Arrhythmias 101

Arrhythmias 101

The Ultimate Easy-to-Read Introductory Book on Arrhythmias

Everything You Need to Know to Get Started Understanding, Recognizing, Diagnosing, and Treating Arrhythmias

Glenn N Levine MD FAHA FACC

Professor of Medicine
Baylor College of Medicine
Director, Cardiac Care Unit
Michael E DeBakey VA Medical Center
Houston, Texas, USA

JAYPEE BROTHERS MEDICAL PUBLISHERS (P) LTD

New Delhi • London • Philadelphia • Panama

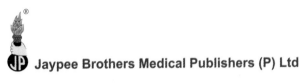

Jaypee Brothers Medical Publishers (P) Ltd

Headquarters

Jaypee Brothers Medical Publishers (P) Ltd
4838/24, Ansari Road, Daryaganj, New Delhi 110 002, India
Phone: +91-11-43574357
Fax: +91-11-43574314
Email: jaypee@jaypeebrothers.com

Overseas Offices

J.P. Medical Ltd
83 Victoria Street, London
SW1H 0HW (UK)
Phone: +44-2031708910
Fax: +02-03-0086180
Email: info@jpmedpub.com

Jaypee-Highlights Medical Publishers Inc
City of Knowledge, Bld. 237, Clayton
Panama City, Panama
Phone: + 507-301-0496
Fax: + 507-301-0499
Email: cservice@jphmedical.com

Jaypee Brothers Medical Publishers Ltd
The Bourse
111 South Independence Mall East
Suite 835, Philadelphia, PA 19106, USA
Phone: + 267-519-9789
Email: joe.rusko@jaypeebrothers.com

Jaypee Brothers Medical Publishers (P) Ltd
17/1-B Babar Road, Block-B, Shaymali
Mohammadpur, Dhaka-1207, Bangladesh
Mobile: +08801912003485
Email: jaypeedhaka@gmail.com

Jaypee Brothers Medical Publishers (P) Ltd
Shorakhute
Kathmandu, Nepal
Phone: +00977-9841528578
Email: jaypee.nepal@gmail.com

Website: www.jaypeebrothers.com
Website: www.jaypeedigital.com

Arrhythmias 101

First Edition: **2013**

ISBN : 978-93-5090-499-2

Printed at: Ajanta Offset & Packagings Ltd., New Delhi

Dedicated to

In the preface to this book, I discuss the importance of being able to diagnose arrhythmias in order to treat and save the lives of patients. I would like to use the dedication of this book to acknowledge and thank all those volunteers and organizations involved in saving the lives of abandoned, abused, and stray animals, particularly those involved with rescue organizations. There is nothing more gratifying than giving a loving home to a rescue dog, and nothing more rewarding than the love and affection that dog gives back to you.

"We can judge the heart of a man by his treatment of animals."

—Immanuel Kant

"The greatness of a nation and its moral progress can be judged by the way its animals are treated."

—Mahatma Gandhi

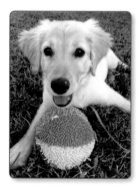

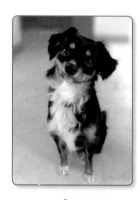

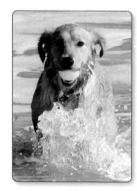

Sadie
Adopted from
Happily Ever After Dog Rescue

Coco
Adopted from
Brazoria County Humane Society

Gabby
Adopted from
Golden Retriever Rescue of Houston

PREFACE

The book *Arrhythmias 101* has been written with the goal of making it the most easy-to-read and understandable introductory book on understanding, recognizing, diagnosing arrhythmias. All healthcare professionals, be they physicians, nurses, physician assistants, or emergency medical personnel, will at some points have to care for the patients who develop arrhythmia. The goal of this book is to give you enough of an understanding of arrhythmias that you can recognize what the arrhythmia is and initiate, when indicated, treatment of the patient. The 13 simple chapters in this book are designed to allow you to quickly and easily achieve this goal.

In addition to the basics of arrhythmia causes and treatment, I have included throughout the book some additional information useful to many readers in the form of "clinical pearls". This information is designed to give the interested reader some extra information on arrhythmias which may be interesting and useful to them.

I have used much of the information, illustrations, and methods of arrhythmia diagnoses contained in this book in the many lectures I have given over the last 15 years to medical students and residents, internists, nurses, physician assistants, and other healthcare professionals. I hope the book proves as useful to you as the information contained in it has been to me in teaching our current and future healthcare professionals. I welcome comments and suggestions from readers.

Thanks to Dr Irakli Giorgberidze for his review of this book and expert suggestions.

Glenn N Levine

CONTENTS

Chapter 1   Normal Depolarization of the Heart   1

Chapter 2   Abnormal Depolarization of the Heart and Arrhythmias   4

Chapter 3   Introduction to Tachyarrhythmias   8

Chapter 4   Tachyarrhythmias Originating in the Atria   11
     Sinus Tachycardia 11
     Atrial Tachycardia 12
     Multifocal Atrial Tachycardia 15
     Atrial Flutter 17
     Atrial Fibrillation 19

Chapter 5   Tachyarrhythmias that Involve the Atrioventricular Node   23
     Junctional Tachycardia 23
     Atrioventricular Nodal Reentrant Tachycardia 26
     Atrioventricular Reentrant Tachycardia 28

Chapter 6   Tachyarrhythmias Originating in the Ventricles   32
     Ventricular Tachycardia 32
     Torsades de Pointes 35
     Ventricular Fibrillation 36

Chapter 7 **Diagnosing Tachyarrhythmias**   38
Narrow Complex Regular Tachycardias 41
Narrow Complex Irregular Tachycardias 46
Wide Complex Tachycardias 48

Chapter 8 **Bradyarrhythmias and Heart Block**   55
Sinus Bradycardia 55
Junctional Rhythms 57
First Degree Heart Block 59
Mobitz Type I Second Degree Heart Block 59
Mobitz Type II Second Degree Heart Block 61
Third Degree (Complete) Heart Block 62

Chapter 9 **Diagnosing Bradyarrhythmias**   66

Chapter 10 **Paced Rhythms**   70

Chapter 11 **Miscellaneous Arrhythmias**   75

Chapter 12 **Basic Life Support and Advanced Cardiac Life Support Treatment of Arrhythmias**   81
Ventricular Fibrillation and Pulseless Ventricular Tachycardia 81
Tachycardia with Pulse 85
Bradycardia with Pulse 90

Chapter 13 **Summary**   92

Index   *95*

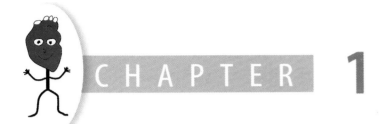

CHAPTER 1

Normal Depolarization of the Heart

Before we can discuss arrhythmias, we need to briefly review the parts of the heart that are involved in the normal depolarization of the heart. Depolarization of the heart begins in the **sinoatrial node**, or **SA node** for short, which is located in the right atrium of the heart. The SA node spontaneously depolarizes, generating a depolarization impulse that travels down the heart and depolarizes the heart. The SA node normally spontaneously depolarizes 60–100 times a minute, leading to the normal heart rate of 60–100 beats per minute. The rhythm that results from normal depolarization of the heart is called **normal sinus rhythm**.

After the SA node depolarizes, the depolarization impulse travels down and across the atria, depolarizing the right and left atria, and arrives at the **AV node**. The impulse is briefly delayed in the **AV node**, contributing to the delay between the P wave and the QRS complex (this distance on the ECG you may remember is denoted as the PR interval).

Once the depolarization impulse passes through the AV node, it then makes its way into and throughout the ventricles. The depolarization impulse first passes through specialized cells called the **His bundle** (or "**Bundle of His**"), which is located near the junction of the atria and ventricles. The depolarization impulse then travels down the **left bundle branch (LBB)** and the **right bundle branch (RBB)** into the ventricles.

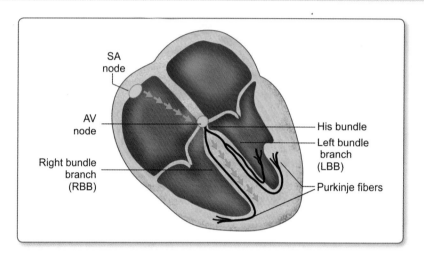

Figure 1.1 Normal depolarization of the heart. Spontaneous depolarization of the SA node leads to a depolarization impulse traveling down the atria to the AV node. The depolarization impulse then travels through the His bundle and down the left bundle branch (LBB) and right bundle branch (RBB) and is distributed into the cells of the ventricles via the Purkinje fibers. The term His-Purkinje system is used to denote the system of specialized cells that transmit the depolarization impulse into and throughout the ventricles, and includes the His bundle, left and right bundle branches, and the Purkinje fibers

Impulse conduction down the left bundle branch leads to depolarization and contraction of the left ventricle. Impulse conduction down the right bundle branch leads to depolarization and contraction of the right ventricle. The depolarization impulse is then distributed into the cells of the left and right ventricle by specialized cells call **Purkinje fibers**. The term **His-Purkinje system** refers to all the specialized cells that conduct the depolarization impulse into and throughout the ventricles, and includes the His bundle, left and right bundle branches, and the Purkinje fibers.

As we will discuss in the next chapter and other chapters, although the SA node is the normal "pacemaker" of the heart, if spontaneous depolarization of the SA node dramatically slows or stops completely, other parts of the heart and conduction system can assume the role of the hearts' pacemaker. Also, if other parts of the heart begin to abnormally spontaneously depolarize at a rate faster than that of the SA node, then that part of the heart takes over as the heart's pacemaker.

Throughout this book, Heartman will offer clinical pearls on diagnosing and treating arrhythmias. This information will be displayed in highlighted box. While the additional information in these clinical pearls will add to your understanding of arrhythmias, the information contained in these clinical pearls is not necessary for you to obtain a basic understanding of diagnosing and treating arrhythmias.

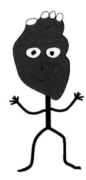

Heartman will offer clinical pearls throughout the book on diagnosing and treating arrhythmias

CHAPTER 2

Abnormal Depolarization of the Heart and Arrhythmias

W hile the SA node is the usual pacemaker in the heart, other tissues in the heart can also spontaneously depolarize, taking over as the pacemaker of the heart. Normally, the depolarization rate of the SA node is faster than the depolarization rate of other tissues. However, on occasion, other tissue in the heart will begin to spontaneously depolarize at a fast rate, faster than the rate of SA node depolarization, and take over as the pacemaker of the heart.

An abnormal and fast heart rhythm is called a **tachyarrhythmia**. There are two basic mechanisms that cause the majority of tachyarrhythmias to occur. One mechanism goes by the fancy term **enhanced automaticity**. When tissue in an area of the heart begins to abnormally depolarize on its own at a fast rate, this phenomenon is referred to as **enhanced automaticity**. Enhanced automaticity is the cause of some arrhythmias we will discuss, including multifocal atrial tachycardia (MAT), junctional tachycardia, most cases of atrial tachycardia, and some cases of ventricular tachycardia. Factors that can lead to enhanced automaticity include mechanical stretch of myocytes (the heart cells), beta-adrenergic stimulation, and hypokalemia.

The other basic mechanism by which many tachyarrhythmias occur is that of a **reentrant circuit.** The term "reentrant circuit" denotes any arrhythmia in which an electrical depolarization impulse repeatedly goes around and around part of the heart, causing an arrhythmia. Reentrant circuits can form in ischemic tissue, infracted (dead) heart tissue, around aneurysms, and even within the AV node. A reentrant circuit can also form in patients who have Wolff-Parkinson-White (WPW) syndrome, in which there is a "bypass tract" (we will explain what a bypass tract is in a later chapter). Reentrant circuits are the cause of some tachyarrhythmias, including AV nodal reentrant tachycardia (AVNRT), AV nodal tachycardia (AVRT), atrial flutter, many cases of ventricular tachycardia (VT), and a few cases of atrial tachycardia. Do not try to memorize all of this now. We will discuss tachyarrhythmias in the next several chapters in greater detail.

Figures 2.1A and B illustrate the two basic causes of most tachyarrhythmias, enhanced automaticity and reentrant circuits. Atrial tachycardia is one of the few rhythms that can be caused by both enhanced automaticity and by a reentrant circuit.

Heartman's Clinical Pearl

A third mechanism that can cause some arrhythmias is called triggered automaticity. Triggered automaticity occurs when a second depolarization impulse occurs prematurely. Triggered automaticity can occur in the setting of excessive adrenergic activity, digitalis toxicity, or high intracellular calcium levels. As triggered automaticity is a rare cause of arrhythmias, this is something that you really do not need to spend time learning about at this point and we will not discuss this rare cause of arrhythmias in this book.

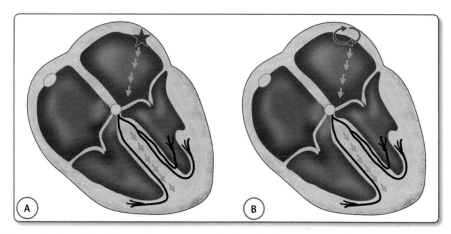

Figures 2.1A and B   The two basic causes of tachyarrhythmias: Enhanced automaticity (A) and reentrant circuit (B)

Bradycardia is defined as any heart rate of <60 beats per minute. **Bradyarrhythmias** (abnormal slow heart rates) may occur if the SA node either stops spontaneously depolarizing completely or depolarizes at a very slow rate. In some cases, another part of the heart may take over as the "pacemaker" of the heart. Bradyarrhythmias may also occur if heart block develops due to dysfunction of the AV node and conduction system. Drugs that can decrease spontaneous depolarization of the SA node and that also slow or block conduction through the AV node include: beta blockers, certain calcium channel blockers (verapamil and diltiazem), digoxin, and many antiarrhythmic agents (such as amiodarone). Medications are not always to blame for dysfunction of the SA node as the heart's pacemaker. The SA node can also become diseased over time, and just lose the ability to spontaneously depolarize at a normal rate. Electrolyte abnormalities and severe hypothyroidism are also causes of bradycardia. We will discuss the causes of bradyarrhythmias more in the chapter on bradyarrhythmias and heart block.

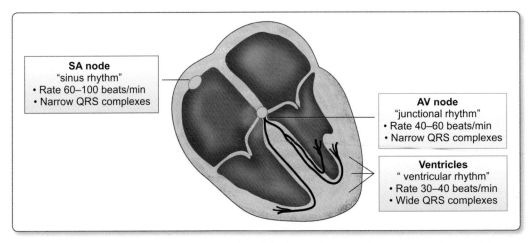

Figure 2.2 If the SA node fails as the pacemaker of the heart, the AV node or tissue in the ventricle may assume the role of the hearts "pacemaker"

If the SA node becomes diseased or is slowed by medications, two other areas of the heart may assume the duty of pacemaker of the heart. One area is the AV node. If the AV node takes over as the pacemaker of the heart, the rhythm is called a **junctional rhythm**, since the AV node is located near the junction of the atria and the ventricles. Depolarization of the AV node usually occurs at a rate of 40-60 beats per minute. Depolarization impulses produced by the AV node travel down the His-Purkinje system, so there is normal depolarization of the ventricles, resulting in a narrow QRS complex. Thus, junctional rhythms usually occur at a rate of 40–60 beats per minute and produce a narrow QRS complex.

If both the SA node and AV node fail as pacemakers of the heart, or if heart block occurs, tissue in the ventricles may assume the role of pacemaker of the heart (Figure 2.2). The usual rate of spontaneous depolarization of this ventricular tissue is 30-40 beats per minute. Since the wave of depolarization initiated by depolarization of this ventricular tissue spreads slowly across the ventricles cell to cell, instead of via the His-Purkinje system, the resulting QRS complex is wide. Thus a ventricular rhythm will usually appear as wide QRS complexes at a rate of 30–40 beats per minute. These slow rhythms that result from spontaneous depolarization of the ventricles are called **ventricular rhythms**. Importantly, spontaneous depolarization of ventricular tissue does not always occur, and if neither the SA node nor AV node is able to spontaneously depolarize, or there is high degree heart block, the patient may develop **asystole** (meaning there is no contraction of the ventricles). That is not good! We will discuss this further in the chapter on bradyarrhythmias and heart block.

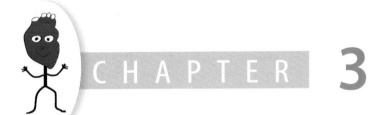

CHAPTER 3

Introduction to Tachyarrhythmias

A **tachycardia** is by definition any heart rhythm at a rate >100 beats per minute. A **tachyarrhythmia** by definition is any *abnormal* heart rhythm that leads to a heart rate greater than 100 beats per minute. In simplest terms, tachycardias are classified as either **supraventricular tachycardias** or **ventricular tachycardias**. Any tachycardia that is caused by a rhythm abnormality originating in the atria or involving the AV node is called a **supraventricular** ("above the ventricle") arrhythmia, or **SVT** for short. Tachycardias that develop in the ventricle are called **ventricular tachycardias**, or **VT** for short.

In the following 3 chapters, we will review the different heart rhythms that cause tachycardias and tachyarrhythmias. We will start at "the top" of the heart in the atria and work our way down to the ventricles. Tachycardias and tachyarrhythmias that occur in the atria include:

- Sinus tachycardia
- Atrial tachycardia
- Multifocal atrial tachycardia (MAT)
- Atrial flutter
- Atrial fibrillation

Tachyarrhythmias that involve the AV node include:

- Junctional tachycardia
- AV nodal reentrant tachycardia (AVNRT)
- AV reentrant tachycardia (AVRT)

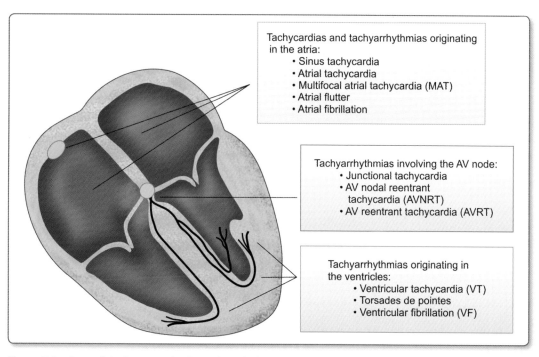

Figure 3.1 Parts of the heart involved in tachyarrhythmias

9

Tachyarrhythmias that originate in the ventricles include:

- Ventricular tachycardia (VT)
- Torsades de pointes (a special type of ventricular tachycardia)
- Ventricular fibrillation (VF)

The accompanying illustration Figure 3.1 demonstrates this useful way of conceptualizing the cause of tachyarrhythmias based upon where in the heart they originate from or what part of the heart they involve. This will hopefully make it easier to understand and remember the different tachycardias, rather than just memorizing a long list of different arrhythmias.

As we discussed in the previous chapter, most tachyarrhythmias that you will encounter are due to one of two basic mechanisms. One mechanism is called **enhanced automaticity**, in which tissue in a part of the heart begins to abnormally depolarize on its own at a fast heart rate. The other common mechanism is a **reentrant circuit**, in which an electrical depolarization impulse repeatedly goes around and around part of the heart. Although there is a third mechanisms that can cause some arrhythmias, called **triggered automaticity**, this is a less common cause of arrhythmias and something you really do not need to spend time learning about at this point.

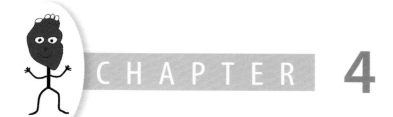

CHAPTER 4

Tachyarrhythmias Originating in the Atria

In this chapter we will discuss the tachycardias that originate in the atria of the heart. Not surprisingly these arrhythmias are called **atrial arrhythmias**. The rhythms we will cover include:

- Sinus tachycardia
- Atrial tachycardia
- Multifocal atrial tachycardia (MAT)
- Atrial flutter
- Atrial fibrillation

SINUS TACHYCARDIA

Although **sinus tachycardia** is not technically an arrhythmia, it is important to briefly discuss sinus tachycardia, as it can be mistaken for a pathological arrhythmia, and because when it occurs, it is important to figure out what is *causing* the sinus tachycardia. Figure 4.1 shows

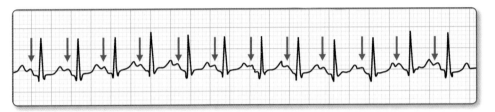

Figure 4.1 Sinus tachycardia. If one does not see there are P waves before each QRS complex, this rhythm could be mistaken for an arrhythmia

an example of sinus tachycardia. If one does not recognize that there are P waves before each QRS complex, this rhythm could be mistaken for a pathological arrhythmia.

Sinus tachycardia is, in general, caused by increased sympathetic stimulation of the SA node in response to some stressor on the body. Stressors that can cause a sinus tachycardia are listed in Table 4.1:

ATRIAL TACHYCARDIA

Atrial tachycardia is an arrhythmia that originates in the right or left atrium at a site other than where the SA node is located. Most commonly, atrial tachycardia is due to a focal area of

Table 4.1: Stressors and other causes in the differential diagnosis of persistent sinus tachycardia

• Anemia	• Hypotension	• Sepsis
• Acute severe bleeding	• Acute MI	• Dehydration
• Hypoxemia	• Heart failure	• Medications and medication overdose
• Pain	• Pericardial tamponade	
• Anxiety	• Tension pneumothorax	• Hyperthyroidism
• Fever	• Pulmonary embolism	

tissue that begins to spontaneously depolarize at an abnormal fast rate (Figure 4.2A). As you may remember, when a part of the heart begins to spontaneously depolarize at an abnormally fast rate we call this **enhanced automaticity**. Atrial tachycardia may also occasionally occur when a **reentrant circuit** develops in the atria (Figure 4.2B). As you may recall, the term "reentrant circuit" denotes any arrhythmia in which an electrical impulse repeatedly goes around and around part of the heart, causing an arrhythmia.

Whether the arrhythmia is caused by enhanced automaticity or a reentrant circuit, the depolarization impulse spreads across the atria, leading to depolarization of the atria. Depolarization of the atria leads to a P wave being

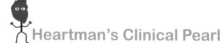

Heartman's Clinical Pearl

Remember, since sinus tachycardia is almost always a physiological response to some stress, one almost never tries to simply treat the tachycardia itself (such as with medications that slow the SA node). Rather, the key in patients with a persistent sinus tachycardia is to identify and treat the underlying cause of the sinus tachycardia.

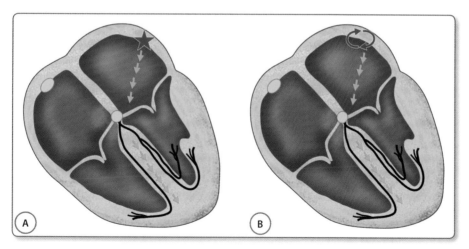

Figures 4.2A and B Atrial tachycardia is usually caused by enhanced automaticity of an area of atrial tissue (A) but on occasion can be due to a reentrant circuit forming in the atria (B)

seen on the ECG (Figure 4.3). However, because the atria are depolarized in a pattern different from that during sinus rhythm, the P waves will appear different in morphology from those seen during sinus rhythm. Depending upon where in the atria the arrhythmia develops, the P waves in some leads may appear inverted (as shown by the arrows in Figure 4.3). Once the depolarization has spread across the atria, the depolarization impulse continues down the AV node and into the ventricles. Depolarization of the ventricles leads to QRS complexes being seen on the ECG. Thus, in atrial tachycardia, we see abnormal or inverted P waves before each QRS complex, as is shown in the below rhythm strip (Figure 4.3).

Although the rate of atrial tachycardia can vary anywhere between 100–250 beats per minute, the heart rate most commonly seen in patients with atrial tachycardia is usually in the range of 160–180 beats per minute. Atrial tachycardia can occur in diseased hearts and in structurally normal hearts. Atrial tachycardia may be caused by digoxin toxicity. Very short runs (< 10–20 beats) of atrial tachycardia are not infrequently seen on Holter monitoring and are often not associated with symptoms, although more sustained episodes may cause symptoms such as palpitations.

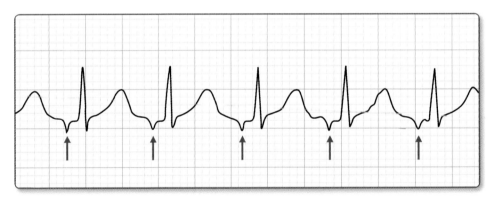

Figure 4.3 The ECG seen with atrial tachycardia. The P wave morphology with atrial tachycardia is different than the P waves that are seen with normal sinus rhythm, and in this case appear "inverted" in this telemetry strip

Atrial tachycardia will usually resolve at some point on its own. Antiarrhythmic agents or other medications are usually not used to try to break the arrhythmia or slow the heart rate, since such drugs rarely acutely terminate the arrhythmia or slow conduction through the AV node. Atrial tachycardia will uncommonly be terminated by administration of adenosine. Since atrial tachycardia is more commonly the result of enhanced automaticity than of a reentrant circuit, cardioverting ("shocking") the patient usually does not terminate the arrhythmia.

MULTIFOCAL ATRIAL TACHYCARDIA

Multifocal atrial tachycardia (or "**MAT**" for short) is an arrhythmia that is caused by multiple sites of tissue in the atria depolarizing at different times (Figure 4.4). Each time one of these sites spontaneously depolarizes, the atria are depolarized. Because these different

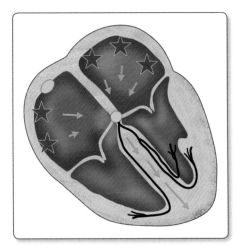

Figure 4.4 Multifocal atrial tachycardia (MAT). There are multiple areas in the atria in which the tissue has begun to spontaneously depolarize

15

areas of depolarizing tissue are spontaneously depolarizing at different times, impulses reach the AV node and are conducted in to the ventricles at varying intervals, leading to an irregular heartbeat.

Because in MAT depolarization of the atria begins at different parts of the atria, the differing patterns of atrial depolarization leads to P waves of different morphologies (arrows in the Figure 4.5). Since spontaneous depolarization of different parts of the atria occurs at different times, the resulting rhythm is irregular (there are varying intervals between the QRS complexes). By definition, MAT is diagnosed when there are at least 3 distinct P wave morphologies and the heart rate is great than 100 beats per minute.

MAT most often occurs in patients with lung disease, particularly those with COPD. The usual "treatment" for MAT is to treat the *underlying cause* that has triggered it, such as a COPD exacerbation. Antiarrhythmic agents or other medications are usually not used to try to terminate the arrhythmia or slow the heart rate. Since the arrhythmia is caused by **enhanced automaticity** of tissues in the atria, "shocking" the patient will not terminate the arrhythmia.

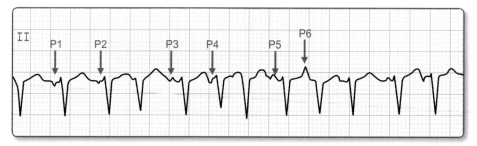

Figure 4.5 The ECG seen with multifocal atrial tachycardia (MAT). The rhythm is irregular and there are numerous P waves of differing morphology before each QRS complex. P1-P6 denote different P wave morphologies

ATRIAL FLUTTER

Atrial flutter is another arrhythmia that occurs in the atria. An impulse travels around and around the atria in a repetitive loop, forming what is called a **reentrant loop** or more technically a **reentrant circuit**. This reentrant circuit is illustrated in Figure 4.6.

In most persons, the impulses travel around the reentrant circuit about 300 times per minute (with a range of 250–350 impulses per minute). Each time the impulse travels around the reentrant circuit, it depolarizes the atria, leading to the "saw tooth pattern" **flutter waves** seen in atrial flutter (Figures 4.7 and 4.8).

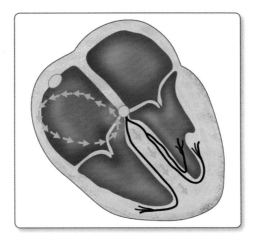

Figure 4.6. Atrial flutter. A reentrant circuit forms in the atria, leading to the arrhythmia

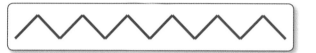

Figure 4.7 The "saw tooth" pattern on the ECG caused by atrial flutter

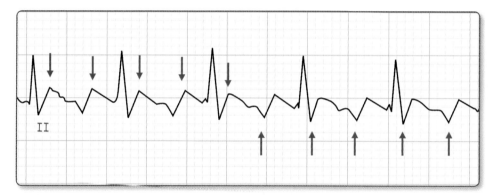

Figure 4.8 The "saw tooth" pattern of flutter waves that are seen in atrial flutter.

The AV node cannot conduct each of these 300 impulses per minute down into the ventricle. Instead, in many persons, it will conduct every other impulse down in the ventricle. When this occurs, we say that there is 2:1 AV conduction, meaning that for every 2 depolarizations in the atria, there is 1 depolarization of the ventricle. Thus, in many people who experience atrial flutter, the actual flutter rate is 300 beats per minute, but the ventricular rate is 150 beats per minute. In some people, if the AV node is "sick" or diseased, or if that person is on medications that slow conduction in the AV node, the AV node will conduct even fewer impulses from the atria down into the ventricle. Such persons may have 3:1 conduction or even 4:1 conduction, leading to ventricular rates of 100 or 75 beats per minute. In other persons, there may be a varying degree of conduction, leading to an irregular ventricular rate. We will discuss this more in a later chapter.

Although atrial flutter occurs in different parts of the atria, it most commonly occurs in the lower part of the right atrium. A wide spectrum of diseases is associated with the occurrence of atrial flutter. Depending on the ventricular response rate, patients may be asymptomatic or may experience symptoms such as palpitations, lightheadedness, shortness of breath, or chest discomfort.

When atrial flutter occurs, there is not the normal, forceful, contraction of the atria. Because of this, patients with atrial flutter are considered to be at risk for forming a clot (more technically called a **thrombus**) in a part of the left atrium called the **left atrial appendage.** Because there is a small chance that such a clot can **embolize** into the circulation and to the brain, patients with atrial flutter are considered to be at risk of having a stroke.

There are two basic approaches to the patient with atrial flutter. If the ventricular response rate is too fast, then the patient can be treated with medications that decrease conduction of impulses from the atria through the AV node into the ventricles. Medications that decrease conduction of impulses through the AV node include **beta blockers** (such as metoprolol, atenolol and carvedilol), certain **calcium channel blockers** (diltiazem and verapamil), and **digoxin**. The other approach is to shock (or more technically electrically **cardiovert**) the patient out of atrial flutter and back into normal sinus rhythm.

Long-term treatment to prevent the recurrence of atrial flutter includes either the use of antiarrhythmic agents or electrical ablation of part of the tissue involved in the reentrant circuit.

ATRIAL FIBRILLATION

Atrial fibrillation is a strange arrhythmia that also occurs in the atria. In atrial fibrillation, multiple "wavelets" of depolarization are constantly forming and reforming in the atria (Figure 4.9). As a result, there is no organized depolarization of the atria, and rather than contract in any organized manner, the atria just "fibrillate". Some of the many impulses generated by these wavelets of depolarization reach the AV node, and some of these are conducted down the atria into the ventricles. Because these depolarization impulses reach the AV node at irregular intervals, and because the AV node conducts some of these impulses down into the ventricle at irregular intervals,

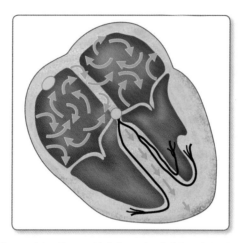

Figure 4.9 The multiple "wavelets" of depolarization impulses in atrial fibrillation

ventricular depolarization and contraction occurs at irregular intervals. Thus, with atrial fibrillation, there is what is called an **irregular ventricular response rate**, similar to what we see with MAT. In some patients with a healthy AV node, the ventricular response rate can be in the range of 150–180 beats per minute. In those with sicker AV nodes or those on medications that decrease conduction through the AV node, the ventricular response rate will be slower.

Because in atrial fibrillation there is no organized depolarization of the atria, there are no P waves seen on the ECG. Rather, there are only numerous, random, and varying small bumps (or deflections) of the ECG tracing. These varying deflections are called **fibrillatory waves** (Figure 4.10).

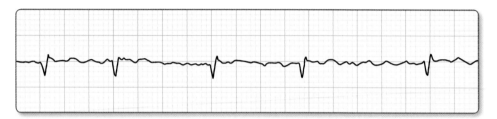

Figure 4.10 The ECG in atrial fibrillation. No P waves or organized atrial activity is evident. The small random deflections of the ECG baseline are due to fibrillatory waves

There are numerous causes of atrial fibrillation. Atrial fibrillation not infrequently occurs in persons with dilated atria and in those with heart failure. Table 4.2 lists some of the important causes of atrial fibrillation to consider when you encounter a patient who has developed atrial fibrillation.

In some patients, atrial fibrillation is believed to be triggered by impulse formation in one of the 4 **pulmonary veins** that drain blood from the lungs to the left atrium. The impulse begins in the pulmonary vein and is then propagated throughout the atria, leading to atrial fibrillation. This impulse initiation and spread is illustrated in Figure 4.11. In such patients, a procedure called a **pulmonary vein ablation** may be performed in order to prevent atrial fibrillation from recurring.

Since there is no organized contraction of the atria, patients with atrial fibrillation are at risk of forming a blood clot ("thrombus") in the part of the atria called the **left atrial appendage**. As with atrial flutter, such patients have a small but real risk of having such a blood clot embolize to the brain, causing a stroke. To decrease the risk of blood clots forming in the left atrial appendage of the heart, patients

Table 4.2: Conditions associated with the development of atrial fibrillation

Dilated atria	Pericarditis
Heart failure and cardiomyopathy	Pulmonary embolism
Acute myocardial ischemia	Hyperthyroidism
Coronary artery disease	Toxins (including alcohol)
Hypertension	

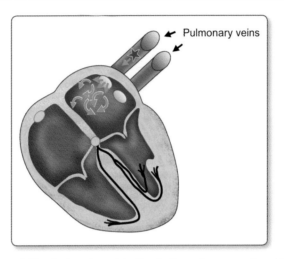

Figure 4.11 An impulse originating in the pulmonary vein, which then spreads through the atria, is the cause of many cases of paroxysmal atrial fibrillation

with atrial fibrillation are often treated with blood thinners such as **warfarin (Coumadin)** or newer blood thinners such as **dabigatran (Pradaxa)**, **rivaroxaban (Xarelto),** and **apixaban (Eliquis).**

As with atrial flutter, there are two basic approaches to the patient with atrial fibrillation. If the ventricular response rate is too fast, the patient is treated with medications that decrease conduction through the AV node, such as **beta blockers**, certain **calcium channel blockers**, and **digoxin**. The other approach to patients with atrial fibrillation is to shock (or more technically electrically **cardiovert**) the patient out of atrial fibrillation and back into normal sinus rhythm. Unfortunately, many patients who develop atrial fibrillation will eventually go back into atrial fibrillation, even if successfully shocked back into normal sinus rhythm.

CHAPTER 5

Tachyarrhythmias that Involve the Atrioventricular Node

In this chapter we will focus on several tachyarrhythmias that involve the atrioventricular (AV) node or tissue in the area of the AV node. The three rhythms we will discuss are:

- Junctional tachycardia
- AV nodal reentrant tachycardia (AVNRT)
- AV reentrant tachycardia (AVNT)

JUNCTIONAL TACHYCARDIA

As we discussed earlier in the book, tissue in the area of the AV node has the potential to spontaneously depolarize. If the SA node fails to spontaneously depolarize, this tissue may take over as the pacemaker of the heart, and such a rhythm, usually occurring at a rate of 40–60 beats/min, is called a "junctional rhythm". It is also possible for this tissue to begin to spontaneously depolarize at a faster rate. If this occurs, and the resulting heart rate is 60–100 beats/min, the rhythm is called "accelerated junctional rhythm". This tissue in the area of the AV node may occasionally begin to depolarize at a rate of >100 beats/min. When this occurs, this spontaneously depolarizing tissue usually takes over the pacemaker function of the heart. The resulting rhythm is called **junctional tachycardia** (Figure 5.1).

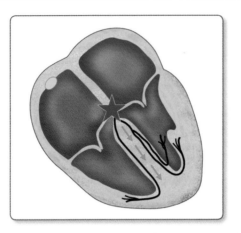

Figure 5.1 Junctional tachycardia. An area of tissue in or near the AV node begins to spontaneously depolarize at a rate > 100 beats/min. Impulses travel from the area of spontaneous depolarization down the His-Purkinje system and into the ventricles

When junctional tachycardia occurs, the resulting ECG shows narrow QRS complexes at a rate of >100 beats/min; P waves are often not present (Figure 5.2).

Unfortunately, different books, review articles, and websites use different terminology when discussing junctional tachycardia. Some sources will use the term "junctional tachycardia" to encompass *any* rhythm that involves the AV node, including the reentrant rhythms discussed below **AV nodal reentrant tachycardia (AVNRT)** and AV **reentrant tachycardia (AVRT).** Also, while some will refer to an arrhythmia due to spontaneous depolarization of the tissue around the AV node as simply "**junctional tachycardia**", others will refer to this as "**ectopic junctional tachycardia**", "**nonparoxysmal junctional tachycardia**", or "**non-reentrant junctional tachycardia**".

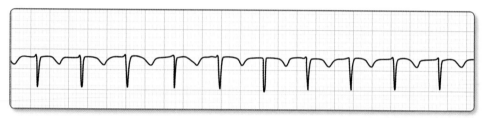

Figure 5.2 Junctional tachycardia. Regular narrow QRS complexes are present at a rate of 120 beats/min. No P waves are present

This is too confusing, and for our purposes in this book we will simply use the term "junctional tachycardia" to refer to a tachyarrhythmia due to abnormal spontaneous depolarization of tissue in or around the AV node, and will separately refer to other arrhythmias that may involve the AV node but involve a reentrant circuit such as AV reentrant tachycardia (AVNRT) or AV reentrant tachycardia (AVRT).

Junctional tachycardia can occur in cases of digoxin toxicity, acute MI, electrolyte abnormalities (such as hypokalemia), after open heart surgery, or due to various other causes. Most commonly, the heart rate is 101–120 beats/min. Much faster (>140 beats/min) narrow complex tachycardias in which there are no P waves or flutter waves present are usually due to either AVNRT or AVRT (discussed below).

Junctional tachycardia usually does not cause the patient significant symptoms. No specific treatment is usually taken in patients who develop junctional tachycardia other than try to determine the underlying cause of the patient developing junctional tachycardia.

Heartman's Clinical Pearl

We name rhythms caused by spontaneous depolarization of the tissue in or around the AV node (located at the "junction" of the heart between the atria and ventricles) by the heart rate:

- Heart rate 40–60 beats/min = junctional rhythm
- Heart rate 61–100 beats/min=accelerated junctional rhythm
- Heart rate >100 beats/min=junctional tachycardia

ATRIOVENTRICULAR NODAL REENTRANT TACHYCARDIA (AVNRT)

AV nodal reentrant tachycardia (Figure 5.3), or simply **AVNRT**, is an arrhythmia that takes place in the area of the AV node. Within the AV node, two impulse-conducting pathways exist. In AVNRT, the impulse goes down one pathway and then up the other in a repetitive loop or circuit. Each time the impulse circles around, an impulse leading to depolarization is sent down the His-Purkinje system into the ventricles.

Each time the impulse circles around the AV node, a depolarizing impulse may also proceed up into the atria, leading to atrial depolarization as well. Atrial depolarization occurs at the same time or just after ventricular depolarization. Because of this, the P waves caused by atrial depolarization are often "buried" in the QRS complex and not seen on an ECG tracing, or P waves are seen occurring at

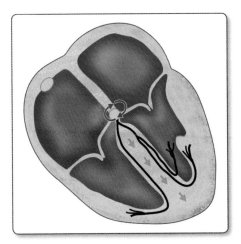

Figure 5.3   AV nodal reentrant tachycardia (AVNRT). A reentrant circuit forms in the area of the AV node

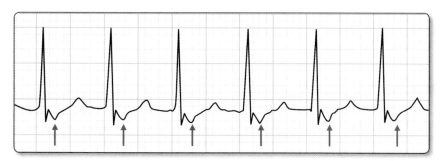

Figure 5.4   An example of AVNRT with small retrograde (inverted) P waves occurring immediately after the QRS complexes

the end of or just after the QRS complex. Because atrial depolarization occurs from the bottom of the atria to the top of the atria, instead of the normal "top to bottom" depolarization, the P waves appear inverted in some leads of the ECG (arrows in Figure 5.4).

Although AVNRT can occur at a rate of anywhere from 120–250 beats per minute, most patients who develop AVNRT will have a heart rate of about 160–200 beats per minute. The most common symptom that patients experience is palpitations. AVNRT can develop in patients without any heart disease, and is a common cause of palpitations in otherwise young and middle aged persons.

AVNRT is not considered to be due to structural heart disease (such as dilated atrial or ventricles) or to ischemic heart disease (coronary artery disease or old myocardial infarction). Rather, it is considered to be simply an electrical disease of the heart. These rhythms are often initiated by **a premature atrial contraction (PAC)** or a **premature ventricular contraction (PVC).**

Initial treatment involves administering medications that slow conduction in the AV node, which can terminate the arrhythmia and prevent its recurrence. **Adenosine** is a short-acting intravenous drug that is frequently used to break AVNRT. Beta blockers and certain calcium channel blockers (diltiazem or verapamil) are used to both break the arrhythmia and to prevent its occurrence. In some patients in whom AVNRT repeatedly recurs, a procedure called **catheter ablation** will be performed.

ATRIOVENTRICULAR REENTRANT TACHYCARDIA (AVRT)

In about 1 to 3 out of every one thousand persons, in addition to the normal conduction system, there is in the heart what is called an **"accessory bypass tract"**. This accessory bypass tract is able to quickly conduct impulses from the atria to the ventricles, bypassing the AV node and His-Purkinje system. The bypass tract can also conduct impulses in the other direction, from the ventricles up into the atria. Patients who have a bypass tract like this are said to have **Wolff-Parkinson-White syndrome** (or simply "**WPW**" for short).

In **AV reentrant tachycardia (AVRT)**, a reentrant circuit can be formed when an impulse goes through the AV node and down the His-Purkinje system into the ventricle, then up the bypass tract into the atria, and then again back down the AV node and His-Purkinje system, forming a repetitive loop or circuit (Figure 5.5). When the impulse in the reentrant circuit travels in this manner, the QRS

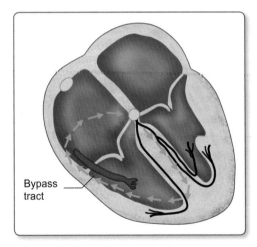

Figure 5.5   In AVRT a bypass tract becomes part of a reentrant loop. Depolarization impulses travel down the His-Purkinje system into the ventricles, then up the bypass tract into the atria, then through the AV node and His-Purkinje system in a repetitive loop. This pattern of impulse conduction is called orthodromic conduction and results in narrow QRS complexes occurring at a regular rate

complexes appear narrow, since ventricular depolarization is occurring via the His-Purkinje system in an organized manner. This pattern of impulse conduction is called "**orthodromic conduction**", though do not worry about memorizing this fancy term unless you really want to.

In AVRT, atrial depolarization occurs after ventricular depolarization. Thus in some cases, P waves can be seen occurring after the QRS complex, often in the ST segment or T wave (Figure 5.6). As in the case with AVNRT, because atrial depolarization is occurring in a "bottom to top" direction, the P waves will appear inverted in some leads. In not all cases of AVRT though will such P waves be visible, and on some rhythm strips all one will see are QRS complexes (Figure 5.7).

Rarely, a reentrant circuit can also be formed in which the depolarization impulse travels from the atria through the bypass track in to the ventricle and then up the His-Purkinje system, through the AV node, and back up to the atria (the reverse direction as described above) This is illustrated in Figure 5.8. The technical term for this type of conduction pattern is called "**antidromic conduction**", though do not bother to try to memorize this fancy term as well unless you really want to! This is a more rare form of AVRT. In this case, because the His-Purkinje system is not involved in depolarizing the ventricles, ventricular depolarization takes longer as the depolarization impulse must travel across the ventricle myocyte to myocyte, and the QRS complexes appear wide. This rare arrhythmia can thus be mistaken for **ventricular tachycardia** (Figure 5.8).

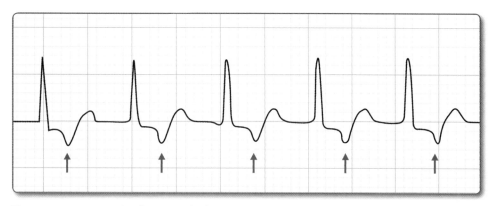

Figure 5.6   An example of AVRT in which retrograde P waves occurring after the QRS complexes are visible. Notice how the inverted P waves distort the ST segments

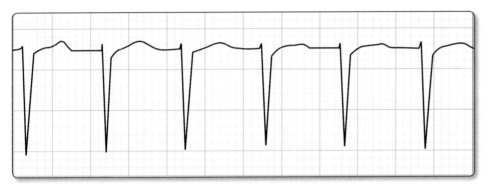

Figure 5.7   An example of a rhythm strip that can be seen in AVRT. In this particular rhythm strip, no P waves are seen

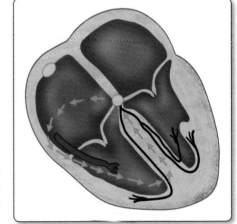

Figure 5.8   A more rare form of AVRT in which impulses travel down the bypass tract and then up the His-Purkinje system and AV node back to the atria. This pattern of impulse conduction is called **antidromic conduction** and results in wide QRS complexes occurring at a regular rate

Like AVNRT, AVRT is considered to be due to a primary electrical problem with the heart, and is not associated with structural or ischemic heart disease. Also like AVNRT, the arrhythmia is often precipitated by a **premature atrial contraction (PAC)** or **premature ventricular contraction (PVC)**.

The heart rate in patients who develop AVRT will most commonly be in the range of 150–220 beats per minute. Like AVNRT, the most common symptom will be palpitations, although some persons may also experience lightheadedness, shortness of breath, or chest discomfort. Also like AVNRT, initial treatment is usually administration of medications that slow conduction through the AV node, which will break the arrhythmia. These medicines include adenosine, beta blockers, and certain calcium channel blockers. Long-term treatment for many patients with WPW syndrome who develop arrhythmias is catheter ablation of the bypass tract.

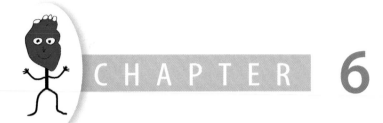

CHAPTER 6

Tachyarrhythmias Originating in the Ventricles

Arrhythmias that originate in the ventricles, called **ventricular arrhythmias**, are the most concerning tachyarrhythmias, as they can lead to hemodynamic collapse and death. The ventricular arrhythmias we will discuss are:

- Ventricular tachycardia (VT)
- Torsades de pointes (a special type of ventricular tachycardia)
- Ventricular fibrillation (VF)

VENTRICULAR TACHYCARDIA

Ventricular tachycardia (often referred to as **VT** or "**V-tach**") is a potentially fatal arrhythmia that originates and occurs in the ventricles. There are several basic mechanisms that can cause VT. One basic cause is that an area of tissue some place in one of the ventricles starts to spontaneously depolarize at a fast rate. As we discussed earlier, this phenomenon is called **enhanced automaticity** (Figure 6.1A). The depolarization impulse generated then spread throughout the ventricles, depolarizing the ventricles. The second basic mechanism that

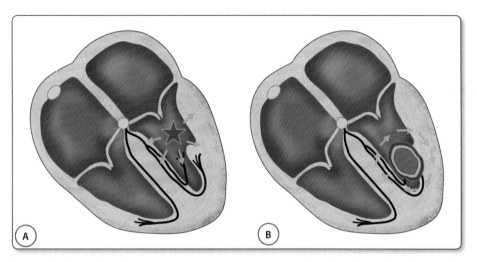

Figures 6.1A and B   VT can be caused by enhanced automaticity (A) or by a reentrant circuit (B)

can cause VT is that depolarization impulse circles around and around part of the ventricle, resulting in a **reentrant circuit** (Figure 6.1B). Such reentrant circuits can form around parts of the ventricles in which there is acute ischemia (such as an acute MI), where there is an old scar from a prior MI, or where there was a prior MI and an aneurysm has now formed.

The risk of ventricular tachycardia is increased in patients with coronary artery disease, with prior MI, and with cardiomyopathy and a depressed left ventricular ejection fraction. The heart rate with VT can be anywhere from the low 100s to 200 beats per minute or more. While in some cases patients may experience only palpitations or lightheadedness, in other patients effective contractions of the ventricles are no longer present and the patient becomes pulseless. "**Stable VT**", in which the patient has only mild symptoms, is usually treated with antiarrhythmic drugs or synchronized cardioversion. "**Pulseless VT**" is a medical emergency and is treated with immediate **defibrillation**. We will discuss the treatment of VT more in the section on BLS and ACLS.

There are several other ways in which VT is classified. One way is classifying the VT based on its duration. **Non-sustained VT** is the term used if the arrhythmia lasts < 30 seconds before self-terminating. **Sustained VT** is if the arrhythmia lasts > 30 seconds.

Another way of classifying VT is based on its morphology. If all the wide QRS complexes look reasonably similar in shape, the VT is called **monomorphic VT** (Figure 6.2). If the morphology of the QRS complexes notably varies, the arrhythmia is called **polymorphic VT** (Figure 6.3). While some patients who develop monomorphic VT are at least relatively stable, patients who develop polymorphic VT are usually unstable and may rapidly become pulseless. Polymorphic VT usually develops in patients with acute myocardial ischemia or in those with prolonged QT intervals.

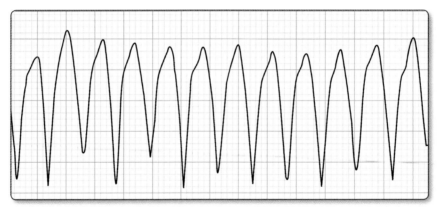

Figure 6.2 An example of monomorphic VT. All the QRS complexes look fairly similar in morphology

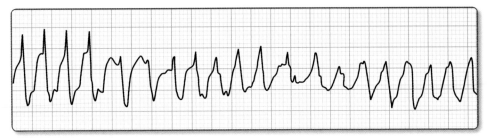

Figure 6.3 An example of polymorphic VT. There is marked variation in the QRS complex morphologies

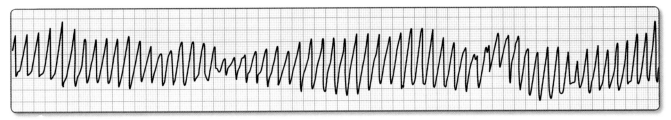

Figure 6.4 Torsades de pointes. A special type of polymorphic ventricular tachycardia in which the imaginary axis of the QRS complexes seems to twist around a point

TORSADES DE POINTES

A special type of polymorphic VT that occurs when the QT interval is prolonged is called **torsades de pointes** (Figure 6.4). The QT interval can be congenitally abnormally prolonged or can be prolonged by drugs such as certain antiarrhythmic agents (procainamide, quinidine, sotalol, dofetilide, amiodarone, ibutilide) or combinations of medicines. Torsades de pointes is a French term that means "twisting of the points". In torsades de points the axis of the QRS complex can be imagined to be changing around a point, as shown in the ECG strip.

Patients who develop torsades de pointes usually become hemodynamically unstable. The arrhythmia can quickly lead to death if not promptly treated with defibrillation.

VENTRICULAR FIBRILLATION

Ventricular fibrillation ("**VF**" or "**Vfib**") is a state in which there is disorganized electrical activity occurring in the ventricles (Figure 6.5). As there is no organized electric activity or ventricular contractions, the patient is pulseless and brain damage and death can rapidly ensue. VF is probably the most common cause of sudden death. Since in VF there is no organized depolarization of the ventricles, normal QRS complexes are not seen. Rather, the disorganized electrical activity is reflected on the ECG by smaller, somewhat random, deflections of the baseline (Figure 6.6).

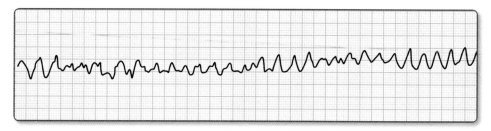

Figure 6.5   Ventricular fibrillation. No discrete QRS complexes are present

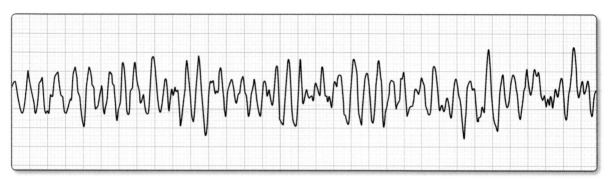

Figure 6.6   Another example of ventricular fibrillation, showing the disorganized electrical activity that occurs with this lethal arrhythmia

VF most commonly occurs in patients with coronary artery disease and may be related in many cases to acute ischemia or acute MI. It also occurs in patients with depressed left ventricular ejection fraction and cardiomyopathies. VF is also associated with electrolyte abnormalities such as hypokalemia. VF may result from untreated ventricular tachycardia, which may degenerate into VF.

The treatment of VF is immediate defibrillation. CPR should be administered while awaiting a defibrillator if one is not immediately available. Treatment of VF is discussed further in the section on BLS and ACLS.

CHAPTER 7

Diagnosing Tachyarrhythmias

Now that we have discussed the major causes of tachyarrhythmias, we are ready to take the next step of discussing how one can diagnose the cause of a tachyarrhythmia seen on an ECG or telemetry monitor. We will use a simple 3 step process to help categorize and diagnose arrhythmias. The three simple steps, which we will discuss in more detail, are:

1. Determine if the QRS complexes seen in the arrhythmia are narrow or wide

2. Determine if the QRS complexes are occurring at regular or irregular intervals

3. Determine if there is any evidence of P waves or atrial activity present

A "narrow QRS complex" is defined as a QRS complex that is < 120 msec in width (< 3 little boxes in width on the ECG strip). A "wide QRS complex" is defined as a QRS complex that is ≥ 120 msec in width (3 or more little boxes in width on the ECG strip). The accompanying illustration (Figures 7.1A and B) shows examples of narrow and wide QRS complexes.

By "regular" we mean that the QRS complexes are all occurring at regular intervals, like the ticking of a clock. In contrast, when the QRS complexes occur at irregular or varying intervals, like the sound of rain droplets falling, we say that the rhythm is **"irregular"**. The accompanying illustration (Figures 7.2A and B) shows examples of QRS complexes that are occurring at regular intervals and QRS complexes that are occurring at irregular intervals.

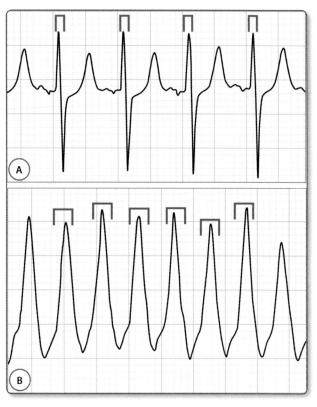

Figures 7.1A and B   Narrow (A) and wide (B) QRS complexes

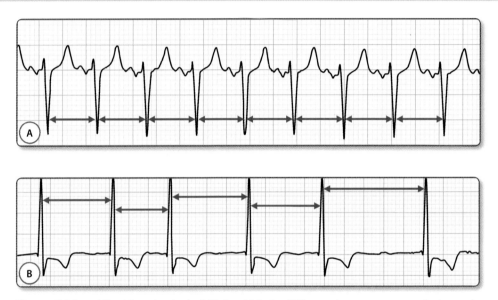

Figures 7.2A and B A "regular rhythm" (A), in which the QRS complexes occur at regular intervals, and an "irregular rhythm" (B), in which the intervals between QRS complexes vary

Based on whether the QRS complexes are narrow or wide, and whether the QRS complexes are occurring at regular or irregular intervals, we can divide tachyarrhythmias into three basic categories:

- Narrow complex regular tachycardias
- Narrow complex irregular tachycardias
- Wide complex tachycardias

Once we have determined if the arrhythmia is a narrow complex regular tachycardia, a narrow complex irregular tachycardia, or a wide complex tachycardia, we can determine the specific rhythm by looking for P waves or atrial activity.

NARROW COMPLEX REGULAR TACHYCARDIAS

There are six rhythms that can cause a narrow complex regular tachycardia:

- Sinus tachycardia
- Atrial tachycardia
- Atrial flutter
- Junctional tachycardia
- AV nodal reentrant tachycardia (AVNRT)
- AV reentrant tachycardia (AVRT)

We can determine which of these rhythms is causing the narrow complex tachycardia by looking for P waves or atrial activity. If there are normal looking P waves before each QRS, the rhythm is simply **sinus tachycardia** (Figure 7.3).

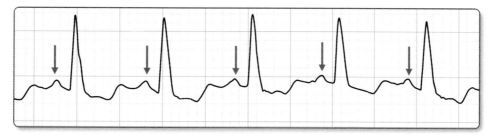

Figure 7.3   Sinus tachycardia. Normal looking P waves (arrows) are present before each QRS complex

If there are abnormal appearing or inverted P waves before each QRS complex, then the rhythm is **atrial tachycardia** (Figure 7.4).

If instead of discrete P waves we see a saw-tooth pattern atrial activity with **flutter waves**, the rhythm is **atrial flutter** (Figure 7.5).

If one sees neither P waves before the QRS complexes nor flutter waves, then the rhythm is either junctional tachycardia, AV nodal reentrant tachycardia (AVNRT) or AV reentrant tachycardia (AVRT). If the rhythm is at a rate of 101–120 beats/min, it is more likely than not the rhythm is junctional tachycardia (Figure 7.6), since AVNRT and AVRT usually result in a faster heart rate than this. If the rhythm is 140 beats/min or more, the rhythm is much more likely to be AVNRT or AVRT than junctional tachycardia. It is usually impossible to determine for sure from the ECG whether the rhythm is AVNRT or AVRT. Statistically, AVNRT is much more common than AVRT, so in most cases the arrhythmia will turn out to be due to AVNRT. However, if the patient has known WPW and a bypass tract, then the rhythm is more likely AVRT.

In both AVNRT and AVRT, discrete P waves may not be visible. In fact, in 80% of cases of AVNRT, any retrograde P waves are buried within the QRS complex and are thus not visible. However, if P waves occurring after the QRS complexes are visible, this may help at least a

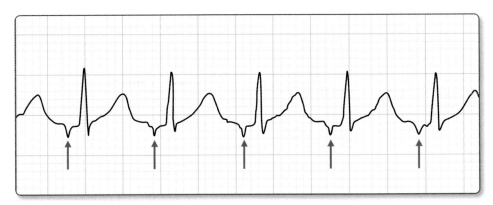

Figure 7.4 Atrial tachycardia. Abnormal looking, inverted P waves (arrows) are present before each QRS complex

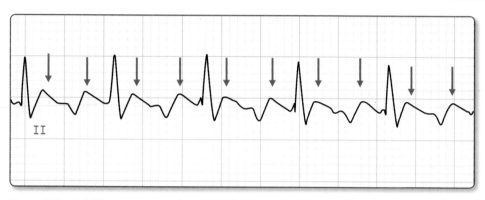

Figure 7.5 Atrial flutter. A saw tooth pattern of atrial activity is present, which is referred to as flutter waves

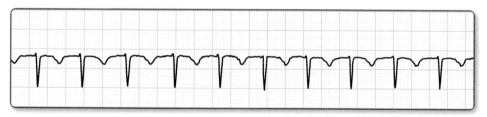

Figure 7.6 Junctional tachycardia. Regular narrow QRS complexes are present at a rate of 120 beats/min. No P waves are present

little in deciding if the rhythm is more likely AVNRT or AVRT. If retrograde P waves are seen at the end of the QRS complex or immediately after the QRS complex, this may make it a little more likely the rhythm is AVNRT, whereas if retrograde P waves are seen a discrete distance from the QRS complexes, this may make it a little more likely the rhythm is AVRT. The following rhythm strips illustrate this concept. It should be noted, however, that there are exceptions to this generalization, and the distance of the retrograde P waves from the QRS complexes cannot be used to definitively decide whether the rhythm is AVNRT or AVRT (Figures 7.7 to 7.9).

In summary, once we determine that the QRS complexes are narrow and are occurring at regular intervals, to determine the rhythm we look for P waves or atrial activity:

- Normal P waves before each QRS complex → sinus tachycardia
- Abnormal or inverted P waves before each QRS complex → atrial tachycardia
- Flutter waves → atrial flutter
- No P waves or retrograde P waves after the QRS complexes → junctional tachycardia, AVNRT or AVRT

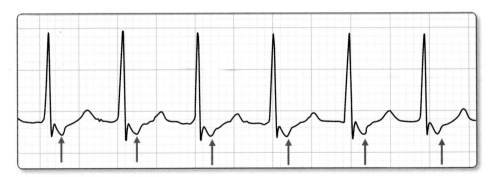

Figure 7.7 In this narrow complex regular tachycardia, retrograde P waves (arrows) are visible immediately after the QRS complexes, making the most likely diagnosis AVNRT

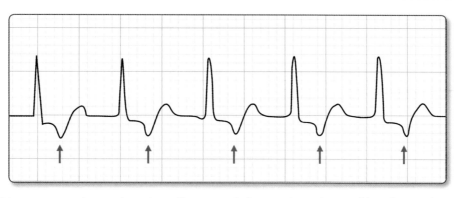

Figure 7.8   In this narrow complex regular tachycardia, retrograde P waves (arrows) are visible a discrete distance after the QRS complexes, making it a little more likely that this arrhythmia is AVRT and not AVNRT

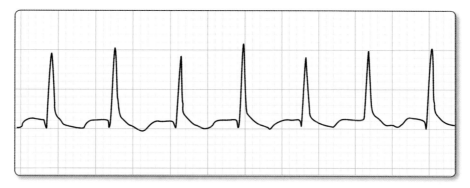

Figure 7.9   In this narrow complex regular tachycardia no P waves or flutter waves are visible before or after the QRS complexes. The rate of 180 beats/min makes this arrhythmia too fast to be junctional tachycardia, and it is either AVNRT or AVRT. Only an electrophysiology (EP) study can determine for sure if the arrhythmia is due to AVNRT or AVRT

NARROW COMPLEX IRREGULAR TACHYCARDIAS

There are three rhythms that can cause a narrow complex irregular tachycardia:

- Multifocal atrial tachycardia (MAT)
- Atrial flutter with "variable" conduction
- Atrial fibrillation.

As we did with the narrow complex regular tachycardias, to determine the cause of a narrow complex irregular tachycardia we will look for P waves or atrial activity. If there are P waves of differing morphologies before each QRS complex, then the rhythm is multifocal atrial tachycardia (MAT) (Figure 7.10).

In the below rhythm strip, flutter waves are clearly visible, making the diagnosis of atrial flutter. Previously, we have seen an example of atrial flutter in which there are 2 flutter waves for each QRS complex, which results from "2:1 conduction" down the AV node. Occasionally, in atrial flutter there is what is called "**variable conduction**" or "**variable block**" of depolarization impulses down the AV node (Figure 7.11). For instance, there may be 2:1 conduction for a couple beats, then 1:1 conduction for a beat, then 3:1 conduction for several

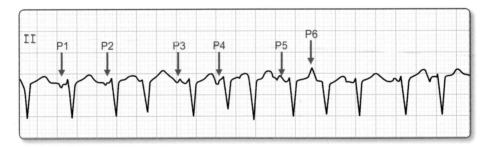

Figure 7.10   Multifocal atrial tachycardia (MAT). There are P waves of differing morphology before each QRS complex. In this example, at least 6 different P wave morphologies (P1-P6) are present

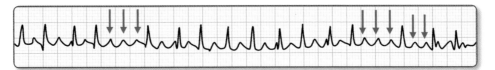

Figure 7.11 Atrial flutter with variable block. There is a varying ratio of flutter waves to QRS complexes, resulting in an irregular rhythm

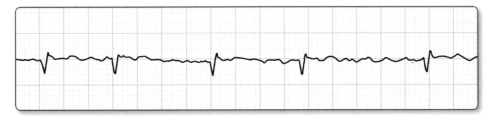

Figure 7.12 Atrial fibrillation. There are no P waves or flutter waves present, only modest random and irregular deflections of the ECG baseline

beats, then more 2:1 conduction. In such cases, instead of QRS complexes occurring at regular intervals, the QRS complexes occur at irregular intervals.

In the example of a narrow complex irregular rhythm below, there are no P waves or ECG signs of organized atrial activity present. The rhythm is, therefore, atrial fibrillation (Figure 7.12). Notice that in atrial fibrillation there can be some modest irregular and random deflections of the ECG baseline, but these deflections should not be mistaken for P waves or flutter waves.

In summary, once we determine that the QRS complexes are narrow and are occurring at irregular intervals, we look for the presence of P waves or atrial activity to determine which of the three possible rhythms are causing the arrhythmia:

- Multiple P waves of differing morphology before each QRS complex → multifocal atrial tachycardia (MAT)
- Flutter waves → atrial flutter
- No P waves or organized atrial activity → atrial fibrillation

WIDE COMPLEX TACHYCARDIAS

There are two basic causes of a wide complex tachycardia:

- Any type of supraventricular tachycardia (SVT) in which there is bundle branch block and the QRS complex is wide
- Ventricular tachycardia (VT)

We need to take a minute to explain what we mean by a **supraventricular tachycardia (SVT)** with **bundle branch block (BBB).** Remember that by "SVT" we are referring to any tachyarrhythmia that does not originate in the ventricles. Thus SVT includes all the arrhythmias we have discussed other than ventricular tachycardia. Both a **right bundle branch block (RBBB)** and a **left bundle branch block (LBBB)** result in a wide QRS complex. Therefore, any combination of SVT and bundle branch block (BBB) will result in a wide complex tachycardia appearing on the ECG. Note that for the purposes of this discussion we will consider sinus tachycardia in the same category as supraventricular tachycardias.

There are several tricks to help determine if a wide complex tachycardia is due to SVT with BBB or due to VT. While a SVT with BBB will usually appear perfectly regular, both In terms of QRS morphology and the RR interval (which is the distance between QRS complexes), VT will often appear slightly irregular. Below is an example of a SVT with BBB. Each QRS complex looks exactly like the others, and the RR intervals are exactly the same. These QRS complexes have been referred to as the "boringly regular" wide QRS complexes seen in an SVT (Figure 7.13).

In contrast, in this example below of monomorphic VT, there is still a slight variation in the QRS morphologies and the RR intervals (Figure 7.14).

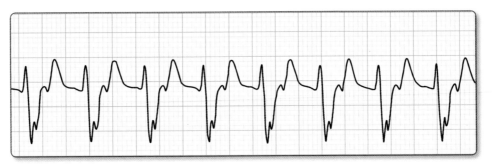

Figure 7.13 The "boringly regular" wide QRS complexes seen in an SVT with BBB

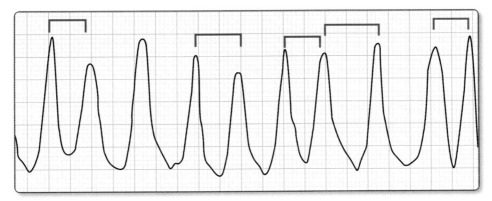

Figure 7.14 In this example of monomorphic VT, the QRS intervals are slightly irregular in morphology and the RR intervals (brackets) are also slightly irregular

Heartman's Clinical Pearl

A rare exception to the above rule is occasionally seen in patients with WPW who develop atrial fibrillation. Patients with WPW who develop atrial fibrillation will have an unusual ECG that shows an irregular rhythm and QRS complexes of varying width. This is because some of the impulses that reach and depolarize the ventricle travel down the AV node and His-Purkinje system, resulting in narrow QRS complexes, while some other impulses that depolarize the ventricle travel down the bypass tract, resulting in wide QRS complexes. Sometimes, impulses traveling down the AV node and His-Purkinje system and impulses traveling down the bypass tract arrive in the ventricle at the same time, resulting in a QRS impulse that is a hybrid of a narrow QRS complex and a wide QRS complex. The resulting rhythm strip is shown below (Figure 7.15), and is essentially a montage of narrow QRS complexes, wide QRS complexes, and QRS complexes of intermediate width. Patients who develop this arrhythmia should not be treated with medications that slow conduction down the AV node, as this may somewhat paradoxically lead to an increase in heart rate as more impulses travel down the bypass tract and depolarize the ventricles, and can lead the patient to develop ventricular fibrillation.

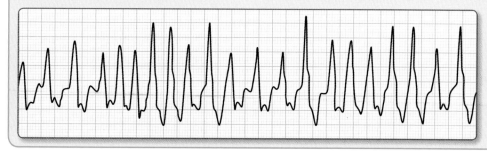

Figure 7.15   An example of atrial fibrillation in a patient with WPW. There is marked variation in the QRS complex morphologies and RR intervals

Perfectly regular wide complex tachycardias are *usually* SVT with BBB, although occasionally a monomorphic VT may look almost perfectly regular. Therefore, the presence of a perfectly regular wide complex tachycardia makes us suspect it is due to an SVT with BBB, but we cannot say for certain this is the case. In contrast, a wide complex tachycardia that is slightly irregular is usually VT.

A second trick to help distinguish SVT with BBB from VT is to look for P waves or organized atrial activity. If we see P waves before each QRS complex, or flutter waves, then we know the rhythm must be some type of SVT with BBB. For example, in the below rhythm strip P waves (arrows) can be seen before each wide QRS complex (Figure 7.16). The rhythm is thus sinus tachycardia.

We also look for P waves any place in the ECG to see if something called **P wave dissociation** in present (Figure 7.17). P wave dissociation (also interchangeably called **AV dissociation**) is a phenomenon that occurs in some patients who develop VT. In such patients, VT develops in the ventricle, depolarizing the ventricle. While this depolarization is occurring in the ventricles, at the same time the SA node in the right atrium may continue to generate impulses which depolarize the atria. Depolarization of the atria and the ventricles occurs independently of each other, hence the term "AV dissociation".

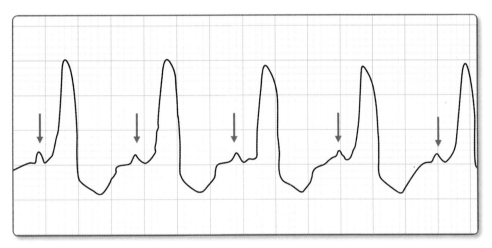

Figure 7.16 Sinus tachycardia with LBBB. Normal looking P waves (arrows) are present before each QRS complex

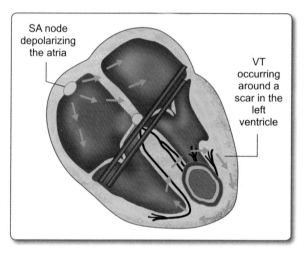

SA node
depolarizing
the atria

VT
occurring
around a
scar in the
left
ventricle

Figure 7.17 "P wave dissociation" ("AV dissociation") occurring during ventricular tachycardia. The atria and ventricles depolarize independent of each other

On the ECG below we see the fast and wide QRS complexes of VT (Figure 7.18). We also may see an occasional P wave, caused by depolarization of the atria. Since the atria and the ventricles are depolarizing at different rates, there is no relationship seen between the P waves and the QRS complexes, hence the term "P wave dissociation" or "AV dissociation". These dissociated P waves may be seen any place on the ECG, including in the ST or T waves. The finding on the ECG of P wave dissociation (AV dissociation) is extremely helpful in making the diagnosis of the arrhythmia, since the finding of P wave dissociate almost always means the wide complex arrhythmia is because of VT.

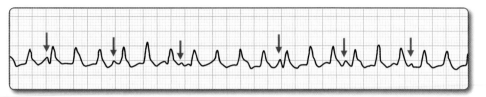

Figure 7.18 An example of P wave dissociation (AV dissociation) occurring in a patient with VT. There is no relationship between the P waves (arrows) and the QRS complexes

In summary, there are several tricks we can use to help distinguish a rhythm caused by SVT with BBB from a rhythm due to VT:

1. Look to see if the QRS complexes are perfectly regular or slightly irregular. If the QRS morphologies and RR intervals (the distance between QRS complexes) are all perfectly the same, then this suggests the rhythm is likely SVT with BBB. If there is slight (or more) variation in the QRS morphologies and RR intervals, then the rhythm is likely VT.

2. Look for P waves or organized atrial activity. If there are P waves before each QRS complex, or flutter waves present, then the rhythm is SVT with BBB. If there is P wave dissociation (AV dissociation), then the rhythm is VT.

Heartman's Clinical Pearl

For the purposes of simplicity, we have stated that a wide complex tachycardia can basically be causes by one of two arrhythmias, either an SVT with bundle branch block or ventricular tachycardia. You may remember, however, that earlier in the book we discussed that in a small percentage (5–10%) of cases of AVRT, the impulse travels down the bypass tract, in to the ventricle, and then up the His-Purkinje system and AV node and in to the atria (Figure 7.19). When this type of reentrant circuit occurs (which we discussed is called antidromic conduction), the resulting QRS complexes are wide (as depolarization across the ventricle occurs slowly). Thus technically, there are three causes of a wide complex tachycardia:

- SVT with bundle branch block
- ARVT with antidromic conduction
- VT

As this is only a very rare cause of a wide complex tachycardia, do not worry if you do not understand this or do not want to spend time memorizing this. This is really something that is important at the level of a cardiologist, but not critical to someone first learning arrhythmia diagnosis and treatment.

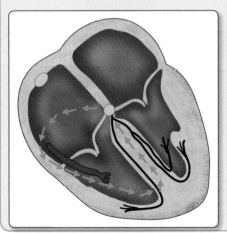

Figure 7.19 A rare form of AVRT in which impulses travel down the bypass tract, across the ventricles, and then up the His-Purkinje system and AV node back to the atria. This pattern of impulse conduction, called antidromic conduction, results in wide QRS complexes occurring at regular intervals

CHAPTER 8

Bradyarrhythmias and Heart Block

In this chapter, we will discuss and review the heart rhythms that can cause a bradyarrhythmia. **Bradycardia** is defined as a heart rate of < 60 beats per minute. A **bradyarrhythmia** is, therefore, any abnormal rhythm that results in a heart rate of < 60 beats per minute. While some cases of bradyarrhythmia are relatively benign, some can be life-threatening, so it is important to be able to identify the cause of the bradyarrhythmia.

SINUS BRADYCARDIA

The normal rate of depolarization of the SA node is 60–100 beats per minute. When the SA node depolarizes at < 60 beats per minute, and the ventricle is thus depolarized at < 60 beats per minute, the resulting rhythm is called **sinus bradycardia** (Figure 8.1).

Numerous conditions and factors can lead to a sinus bradycardia. Some of the most important are listed in Table 8.1. Sinus bradycardia can also be seen in very well conditioned athletes or simply as a normal variant in otherwise healthy persons.

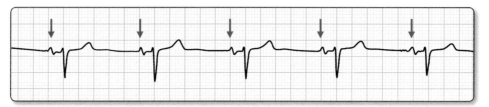

Figure 8.1   Sinus bradycardia. A P wave is present before each QRS complex and the heart rate is < 60 beats per minute

Table 8.1: Causes of sinus bradycardia

Medications that slow depolarization of the SA node (e.g. beta blockers, certain calcium channel blockers, digoxin, antiarrhythmic agents)
Intrinsic SA nodal disease ("sick sinus syndrome", such as can occur in elderly patients)
Hypothyroidism
Electrolyte abnormalities (e.g. hyperkalemia)
Increased vagal tone (such as with an acute inferior wall MI or vasovagal reaction)
Brain injury (stroke or trauma)
Infections that affect the heart
Hypoxemia (low oxygen levels in the blood)

Unless the heart rate is < 40–50 beats per minute or so, patients are rarely symptomatic. In the rare patient who requires treatment for sinus bradycardia, the first step is to address any potential cause, such as discontinuing drugs that slow depolarization of the SA node. In most cases of severely symptomatic bradycardia, acute treatment involves administration of atropine. Temporary transcutaneous pacing is also employed when available in severely symptomatic patients. The acute treatment of symptomatic bradycardia is discussed more in the chapter on BLS and ACLS. Long-term treatment of patients with symptomatic bradycardia is pacemaker implantation.

JUNCTIONAL RHYTHMS

As we have discussed previously, the SA node is able to spontaneously depolarize and acts as the "pacemaker" of the heart. The lower part of the AV node is itself able to spontaneously depolarize, similar to how the SA node spontaneously depolarizes. Since the normal rate of SA node depolarization (60–100 beats per minute) is higher than the rate that the lower part of the AV node spontaneously depolarizes (40–60 beats per minute), the SA node usually acts as the pacemaker of the heart. If however for some reason the SA node either stops spontaneously depolarizing completely or depolarizes at a very slow rate, this lower part of the AV node may take over as the "pacemaker" of the heart. When the AV node acts as the pacemaker of the heart, the rhythm is referred to as a **junctional rhythm,** since it is originating near the junction of the atria and the ventricles (where the lower part of the AV node is located).

The impulses generated by spontaneous depolarizations of the AV node normally travel down the His-Purkinje system into the ventricles, depolarizing the ventricles in the normal manner, and thus the QRS complexes in a junctional rhythm are narrow (Figure 8.2). Since the usual rate of spontaneous depolarization of the AV node is 40-60 beats per minute, the ECG shows narrow QRS

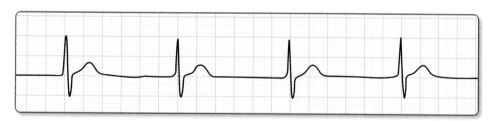

Figure 8.2   Junctional rhythm. There are narrow QRS complexes at a rate of 50 beats/min. No P waves are present before the QRS complexes

complexes usually occurring at a rate of 40–60 beats per minute. In a junctional rhythm, depolarization of the SA node is no longer occurring, and thus normal P waves are usually not preceding each QRS complex, as is illustrated in the accompanying ECG.

While in most cases of junctional rhythm P waves are not present, in some cases P waves may be seen immediately before the QRS complexes (Figure 8.3). This can occur when the depolarization impulse generated by spontaneous depolarization of the AV node travels not only down into the ventricle but also "upward" into the atria, depolarizing the atria "from bottom to top". In such cases, in which spontaneous depolarization of the AV nodal tissue leads to depolarization of the atria and the ventricles, depolarization of the atria and ventricles occur at almost the same time. When this occurs, an often "inverted" P wave may be seen immediately before each QRS complex, as in the below example (Figure 8.3). Note that the visible P wave is very close to the QRS complex, and one should not mistake this for sinus rhythm, in which we expect to see P waves a discrete distance (usually at least 120 msec or 3 "small boxes") before the QRS complexes.

Many persons who develop a junctional rhythm may be asymptomatic. In some, because of the relatively slow heart rate, dizziness, presyncope (the sensation of being about to pass out), mild shortness of breath, fatigue, or decreased exercise ability may develop. Most patients who develop junctional rhythm require no specific acute treatment. Rather, management of such persons usually involves determining why they have developed the junctional rhythm.

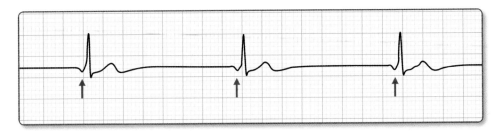

Figure 8.3 Junctional rhythm. In this example, retrograde, inverted P waves (arrows) are visible just before the QRS complexes.

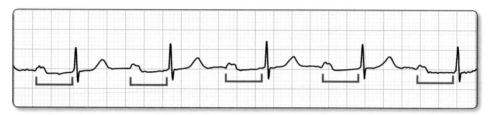

Figure 8.4   First degree heart block, with a prolonged PR interval (brackets). The PR interval is > 200 msec (5 small boxes)

FIRST DEGREE HEART BLOCK

In patients with **first degree heart block,** each impulse generated by the SA node depolarizing is conducted down the AV node and His-Purkinje system in to the ventricles, but conduction through the AV node down into the ventricles is slower than normal. This is reflected in the ECG in that each P wave is followed by a QRS complex, but the PR interval (the distance between the P wave and the QRS interval) is prolonged. By definition, first degree heart block is when the PR interval is > 200 msec (> 5 small boxes on the ECG) (Figure 8.4). First degree heart block in itself does not result in bradycardia. First degree heart block can be caused by medications that slow conduction through the AV node (e.g. beta blockers, certain calcium channel blockers, digoxin, or antiarrhythmic agents), increased vagal tone, or intrinsic disease of the AV node (which can occur with normal aging).

MOBITZ TYPE I SECOND DEGREE HEART BLOCK (WENKEBACH)

Second degree heart block is said to be present when some depolarization impulses generated by depolarization of the SA node are not conducted through the AV node into the ventricle. This results in an ECG in which not all P waves are followed by a QRS complex. When this occurs, we say that there are some "**nonconducted impulses**", "**nonconducted P waves**", or "**nonconducted beats**" present on the

ECG. There are two types of second degree heart block: **Mobitz type I second degree heart block** and **Mobitz type II second degree heart block**. We will first discuss Mobitz type I second degree heart block.

Mobitz type I second degree heart block is usually simply called **Wenkebach**, and we will use that term in our discussion. In patients with Wenkebach, the ECG shows regularly occurring P waves, but the PR interval progressively increases, until there is a nonconducted P wave (a P wave not followed by a QRS complex) (Figure 8.5). What is occurring in the conduction system is that the time it takes the impulse generated by the SA node to travel through the AV node is getting progressively longer and longer until one impulse generated by the SA node simply does not make it down the AV node in to the ventricle at all. After this occurs, and there is a nonconducted P wave, the process begins again, with longer and longer PR intervals until another nonconducted P wave occurs.

Wenkebach often occurs in persons with increased vagal tone, as vagal tone modulates conduction through the AV node. If it also sometimes seen in older patients. Wenkebach may or may not lead to bradycardia, depending on the rate of SA node depolarization and the ratio of conducted beats to nonconducted beats. Wenkebach is often incidentally noted on the telemetry monitor in hospitalized patients who are sleeping, as vagal tone increases during sleep. In itself, Wenkebach rarely causes the patient any symptoms and is a relatively benign rhythm. Although over time the patient may develop other conduction abnormalities, the presence of Wenkebach does not require any specific treatment, and is not an indication for pacemaker implantation.

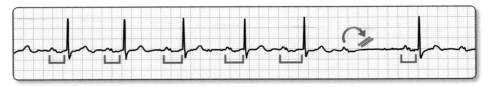

Figure 8.5 Wenkebach. The PR intervals progressively increase until there is a nonconducted P wave or "dropped beat". The brackets show the increasing PR intervals

MOBITZ TYPE II SECOND DEGREE HEART BLOCK

In **Mobitz Type II second degree heart block** (Figures 8.6 and 8.7), there are one or more P waves followed by a QRS complex and then a nonconducted P wave (often called a "dropped beat") in which there is a P wave which is not followed by a QRS complex. In contrast to Wenkebach, in which the PR interval gradually increases until there is a nonconducted P wave, in Mobitz type II heart block the PR interval is constant, and the non-conducted P wave occurs "out of the blue" with no forewarning.

Like Wenkebach, Mobitz type II heart block (Figure 8.7) may or may not lead to bradycardia, depending on the rate of SA node depolarization and the ratio of conducted to nonconducted P waves. Mobitz type II heart block may be due to progressive intrinsic disease within the AV node or acute MI. It is a concerning rhythm, and can progress to complete heart block. Therefore, such patients are hospitalized, placed on telemetry monitoring, and often have either transcutaneous pacing pads placed or a temporary transvenous pacing wire inserted. Permanent pacemaker implantation is usually expeditiously performed in such patients.

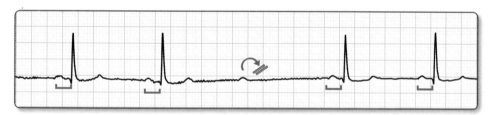

Figure 8.6 An example of Mobitz type II heart block. The PR interval is constant until a nonconducted P wave abruptly occurs

61

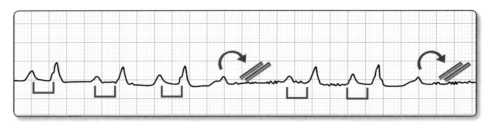

Figure 8.7 Another example of Mobitz type II heart block. The PR interval is constant until a nonconducted P wave abruptly occurs. The nonconducted P waves in this example are present at the end of the T waves (look carefully!)

THIRD DEGREE (COMPLETE) HEART BLOCK

Third degree heart block, which is more commonly referred to as complete heart block, occurs when no P waves are conducted through the AV node down into the ventricle. In such cases, one of three things can occur.

1. As we discussed previously, the lower part of the AV node is itself able to spontaneously depolarize, similar to how the SA node spontaneously depolarizes. If there is complete heart block, this lower part of the AV node may take over as the "pacemaker" of the heart. In cases of complete heart block, when the AV node takes over as the pacemaker of the heart the rhythm is referred to as a **junctional escape rhythm**. These junctional rhythms consist of narrow QRS complexes at a rate usually of 40–60 beats per minute. Since the SA node continues to spontaneously depolarize and depolarize the atria, P waves are seen on the ECG. Since, however, there is complete heart block present, the P waves are not followed by QRS complexes, but rather seem to just "march through" the QRS complexes that occur as a result of the junctional escape rhythm. This is illustrated on the below rhythm strip (Figure 8.8)

2. Some myocardial cells ("myocytes") located in the ventricles are also occasionally able to spontaneously depolarize. If there is complete heart block and there is no junctional escape rhythm, then these myocytes may assume the role of "pacemaker" of

the heart. When there is complete heart block and cells in the ventricle begin to spontaneously depolarize and take over as the effective pacemaker of the heart, the rhythm is called a **ventricular escape rhythm**. The rate of spontaneous depolarization of ventricular cells is usually 30–40 beats per minute. Since depolarization of the heart begins in the ventricles, depolarization impulses have to spread cell to cell, instead of using the much faster His-Purkinje system to spread the depolarization impulse. This results in a wide QRS complex. Therefore, in patients with complete heart block and a ventricular escape rhythm, there are usually wide QRS complexes at a rate of 30–40 beats per minute. An example of complete heart block with a ventricular escape rhythm is shown in the below ECG tracing (Figure 8.9).

3. The third thing that can occur when there is complete heart block is that there is complete heart block with neither a junctional escape rhythm nor a ventricular escape rhythm. In such cases, there is **asystole** and imminent death (Figure 8.10).

Causes of complete heart block include medication effects or frank overdose (e.g. beta blockers, calcium channel blockers, digoxin, or antiarrhythmic agents), progressive intrinsic disease of the AV node, and acute MI.

Complete heart block is always an indication for admission, telemetry monitoring, and intermediate or intensive care monitoring. At a minimum, transcutaneous pacing pads are usually placed on the patient. A temporary transvenous pacing wire may be placed in

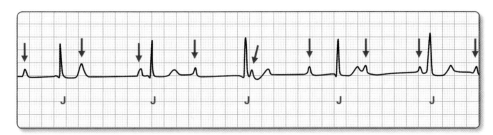

Figure 8.8 Complete heart block with a junctional escape rhythm. The P waves (arrows) are not conducted and there is a narrow QRS complex junctional escape rhythm ("J")

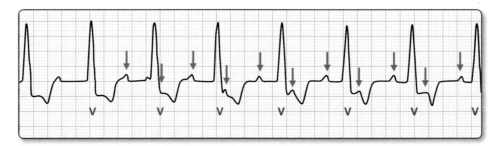

Figure 8.9 Complete heart block with a ventricular escape rhythm. The P waves (arrows) are not conducted and appear to "march through" the QRS complexes. The wide QRS complexes ("V") are ventricular beats due to a ventricular escape rhythm

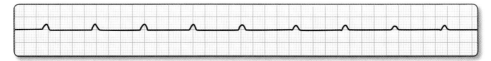

Figure 8.10 Complete heart block with asystole. Only P waves are visible and no QRS complexes are present. There is neither a junctional or ventricular escape rhythm

cases of higher concern that the patient may develop asystole. A junctional escape rhythm is considered more "stable" than a ventricular escape rhythm. That is, the patient is considered to be less likely to suddenly develop asystole than when there is a ventricular escape rhythm (a ventricular escape rhythm is considered an unreliable escape rhythm). Unless a reversible cause of the complete heart block is identified and can be easily treated (such as digoxin overdose), the patient is expeditiously treated with permanent pacemaker implantation.

Bradyarrhythmias and Heart Block

Heartman's Clinical Pearl

It is sometimes confusing to those learning arrhythmia diagnosis whether an arrhythmia is because of complete heart block or due to some type of tachyarrhythmia. The key in deciding which of these two causes of the abnormal heart rhythm is comparing the rate of the P waves with the rate of the QRS complexes. In complete heart block, one will always see on the rhythm strip P waves occurring at a rate *faster* than the QRS complexes that result from either the junctional escape rhythm or the ventricular escape rhythm. Put more simply, one will see more P waves than QRS complexes. These P waves will have no fixed relationship to the QRS complexes, since impulses from the SA node and atria are not being conducted down the AV node. In contrast in a tachyarrhythmia in which there is abnormal spontaneous depolarization of the AV node (resulting in a junctional tachycardia), a reentrant rhythm such as AVNRT or AVRT, or abnormal spontaneous depolarization of the ventricle (resulting in ventricular tachycardia), the P wave rate will either be *slower than or similar to* the QRS complex rate. In other words, there will be either more QRS complexes than P waves (such as can occur with ventricular tachycardia and P wave dissociation) or a similar number of P waves and QRS complexes (which may occur with junctional tachycardia, AVNRT, or AVRT).

65

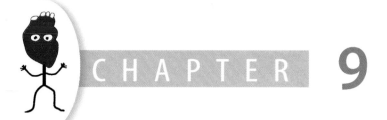

CHAPTER 9

Diagnosing Bradyarrhythmias

Now that we have discussed the causes of bradyarrhythmias, we can set about discussing how to diagnose the cause of a bradyarrhythmia. Similar to how we set about diagnosing the cause of a tachyarrhythmia, the key step in determining the rhythm in patients with bradycardia is looking for P waves.

If normal appearing P waves are seen occurring a normal distance before each QRS complex, the rhythm is **sinus bradycardia**, as in Figure 9.1.

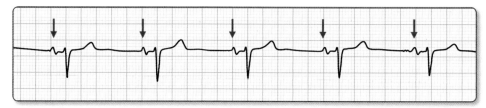

Figure 9.1   Sinus bradycardia. A P wave (arrows) is seen before each QRS complex and the heart rate is < 60 beats/min

If no P waves are seen before each QRS complex, or inverted P waves are seen immediately before the QRS complex, and the QRS complexes are narrow, then the rhythm is a **junctional rhythm** (Figure 9.2). Remember that junctional rhythms usually occur at a rate of 40-60 beats per minute.

If some P waves are followed by a QRS complex, but some other P waves are not followed by a QRS complex, then the rhythm is **second degree heart block**. If the PR interval progressively increases before the nonconducted P wave, then the rhythm is **Mobitz type I second degree heart block (Wenkebach)** (Figure 9.3).

If instead there are constant PR intervals and then a nonconducted P wave suddenly occurs, the rhythm is **Mobitz type II second degree heart block** (Figure 9.4).

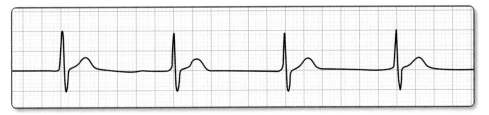

Figure 9.2   Junctional rhythm. No P waves are present before each QRS complex and the QRS complexes are narrow and occurring at a rate of 50 beats/min

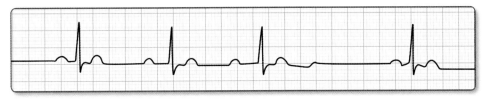

Figure 9.3   Mobitz type I second degree heart block (Wenkebach). The PR interval progressively increases until there is a nonconducted P wave

67

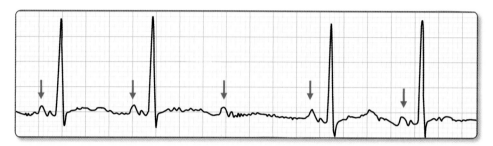

Figure 9.4 Mobitz type II second degree heart block. The PR interval is constant until there is "out of the blue" a nonconducted P wave

 Heartman's Clinical Pearl

Occasionally, you will come across a rhythm in which every other P wave is nonconducted (such as the below rhythm strip) (Figure 9.5). Because there is only one conducted P wave before there is a nonconducted P wave, we cannot tell if the PR interval is progressively increasing or not before there is a nonconducted P wave, and therefore cannot say whether this is Mobitz type I heart block (Wenkebach) or Mobitz type II heart block. We usually just call such rhythms "2:1 AV block".

Patients with acute inferior MI not infrequently develop second degree heart block with this pattern of every other P wave being nonconducted. Inferior MI often leads to increased vagal tone, and in most such patients the cause of this heart block turns out to be Wenkebach, which, as we discussed, is often caused by increased vagal stimulation of the AV node. In contrast, in patients with acute anterior MI, the arrhythmia is often due to Mobitz type II heart block, and suggests damage to the conduction system and the need for pacemaker placement.

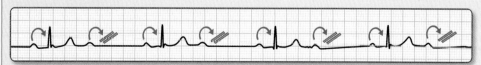

Figure 9.5 Second degree heart block in which every other P wave is not conducted

If P waves are present, are occurring at a rate faster than the QRS complexes, and are "marching through" the QRS complexes (have no fixed relationship to the QRS complexes), then the rhythm is **third degree (complete) heart block**. If narrow complex QRS complexes are present, usually at a rate of 40–60 beats per minute, then the rhythm is **complete heart block with a junctional escape rhythm** (Figure 9.6).

If wide QRS complexes are present, usually at a rate of 30–40 beats per minute, the rhythm is **complete heart block with a ventricular escape rhythm** (Figure 9.7).

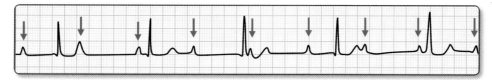

Figure 9.6 Third degree (complete) heart block with a junctional escape rhythm. The P waves (arrows) appear to just "march through" the QRS complexes. Narrow QRS complexes are present at a rate of about 40 beats per minute

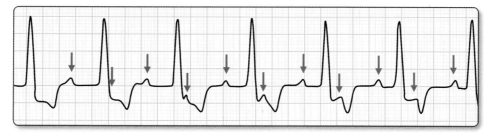

Figure 9.7 Third degree (complete) heart block with a ventricular escape rhythm. The P waves (arrows) appear to just "march through" the QRS complexes. Wide QRS complexes are present due to the ventricular escape rhythm

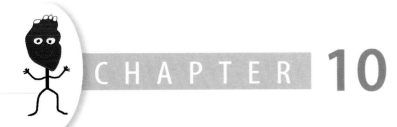

CHAPTER 10

Paced Rhythms

Paced rhythms can often appear on first glance as arrhythmias, both bradyarrhythmias and tachyarrhythmias. It is, therefore, important to be familiar with paced rhythms and how to recognize them.

Pacemakers are usually implanted if either the SA node is dysfunctional and the heart rate is too slow, or the AV node and conduction system become diseased and fail to normally conduct depolarization impulses into the ventricles. In most patients, a pacemaker lead is placed in both the right atrium and in the right ventricle (Figure 10.1). These leads serve two functions. The leads serve to allow the pacemaker to monitor the heart rhythm and determine if it needs to pace the atria and/or the ventricles. The leads also serve to deliver when needed electrical depolarization impulses to the atria and/or ventricles, initiating depolarization of the atria and/or ventricles.

The way most modern pacemakers work is as follows. First, the pacemaker lead in the right atrium waits a programmed amount of time, waiting to see if it senses a depolarization impulse generated by the SA node. If it does, then the pacemaker realizes there is no need for it to generate a depolarization impulse itself. If it does not sense a native depolarization impulse and P wave, then the pacemaker goes ahead and generates a depolarization impulse. Whether the SA node generates a depolarization impulse or the pacemaker does this, the pacemaker then waits to see if the pacemaker lead in the right ventricle detects that the depolarization impulse has successfully made it down the AV node and His-Purkinje system into the ventricles. If it does detect that the depolarization impulse has made it down into the

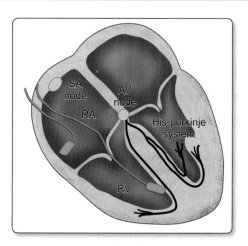

Figure 10.1 Pacemaker leads present in the right atrium (RA) and right ventricle (RV)

ventricles, then it does not itself generate a depolarization impulse. If it does not sense that the depolarization impulse has made it down into the ventricle, then it generates a depolarization impulse itself.

When the pacemaker generates a depolarization impulse, it appears on the ECG as a small vertical spike. It is important to become familiar with recognizing such pacemaker spikes so that a rhythm is not mistakenly identified as a bradyarrhythmia or tachyarrhythmia. We will see examples of these pacemaker spikes in the ECGs below (Figure 10.2).

In some persons, the primary problem is a dysfunctional SA node. The AV node continues to be able to conduct impulses into the ventricle. In such patients, the pacemaker paces the atria only. As shown below, the ECG demonstrates an atrial pacing spike (arrow) a distance before each QRS complex (Figure 10.2). P waves are present immediately after the pacing spike. This rhythm is termed an **atrial paced rhythm**. Notice that the P waves in atrial paced rhythms are generally smaller and harder to see than the normal P waves seen in sinus rhythm.

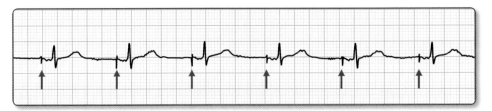

Figure 10.2 Atrial paced rhythm. Pacing spikes (arrows) and subtle P waves generated by the pacemaker depolarization impulses are present before each QRS complex

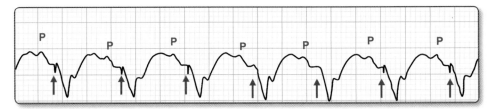

Figure 10.3 Ventricular paced rhythm. P waves (P) are followed by ventricular pacing spikes (arrows) and QRS complexes generated by the pacemaker depolarization impulses

In other persons, the primary problem is an AV node and conduction system that cannot conduct depolarization impulses into the ventricle. In these patients, the pacemaker is able to sense that the SA node has generated a depolarization impulse but that depolarization impulse has not been conducted down in the ventricle. The pacemaker, therefore, paces the ventricle after each atrial depolarization. As shown above, the ECG demonstrates a sinus tachycardia with pacer spikes immediately before each QRS complex (Figure 10.3). The pacemaker is sensing that there is a sinus tachycardia, and is pacing the ventricle at that rate. Note that paced QRS complexes are wide, since the His-Purkinje system is not involved in depolarizing the ventricle and depolarization impulses generated by the pacemaker lead spread slowly across the ventricles. Notice in the below rhythm strip that if one did not notice that there were P waves are pacing spikes it would be easy to mistake this rhythm for a wide complex tachycardia (Figure 10.3).

The below tracing is another example of a ventricular paced rhythm. Notice again that if you did not recognize that there were ventricular pacing spikes present one could easily mistake this rhythm as a wide complex tachycardia (Figure 10.4).

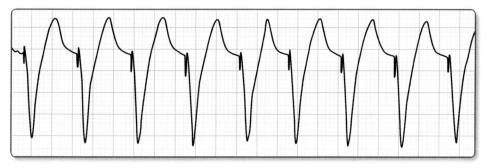

Figure 10.4   This ventricular paced rhythm could be mistaken for a wide complex tachycardia unless the pacer spikes immediately before the QRS complexes are noticed

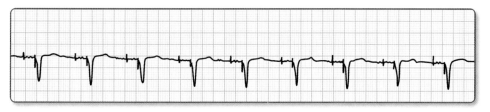

Figure 10.5   AV sequential pacing. There are both atrial and ventricular pacing spikes present

Figure 10.5 is an example of **AV sequential pacing**. AV sequential pacing means that both the atria and ventricles are paced, with an atrial pacing impulse followed shortly thereafter by a ventricular pacing impulse. Both an atrial pacing spike and a ventricular pacing spike are present for each beat (note you have to look carefully to see the ventricular pacing spikes, which is often the case!). The pacemaker is thus pacing both the atria and the ventricles (hence the name AV sequential pacing).

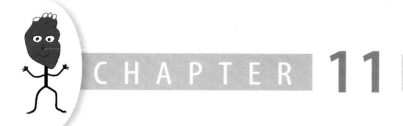

CHAPTER 11

Miscellaneous Arrhythmias

We have now covered the basics of arrhythmias. We will now briefly discuss a few other arrhythmias and ECG tracings that you will likely encounter while taking care of patients, and thus should be able to recognize.

The below ECG is an example of what is called **tachy-brady syndrome** (Figure 11.1). The ECG shows that the patient initially has a fast heart rate due to atrial fibrillation. Midway through the ECG strip the atrial fibrillation terminates. There is a several second pause

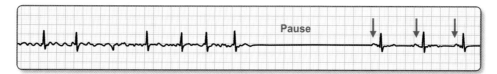

Figure 11.1   An example of tachy-brady syndrome (sick sinus syndrome). When the atrial fibrillation terminates, there is a several second pause before normal sinus rhythm resumes (Reproduced with permission from Levine GN and Podrid PJ. The ECG Workbook. John Wiley and Sons)

until normal sinus rhythm resumes. Tachy-brady syndrome is an occasional cause of syncope, particularly in older patients. Such patients have paroxysmal atrial fibrillation (atrial fibrillation that spontaneously begins and spontaneously terminates). When the atrial fibrillation terminates, there is a several second pause before normal sinus rhythm resumes. If this pause is more than 3 or 4 seconds, the patient may experience lightheadedness or even overt syncope. This condition is often referred to as **sick sinus syndrome**, although tachy-brady syndrome is a better and more precise way to describe the arrhythmia and condition. Patients with tachy-brady syndrome often require placement of a permanent pacemaker.

The below rhythm is an example of **atrial tachycardia with high degree AV block**, which is an arrhythmia that can occur with digoxin toxicity (Figure 11.2). There are unusual P waves occurring at a rate of 180 beats per minute. Only one out of every 4 of these P waves appears to be conducted through the AV node, leading to ventricular depolarization and a QRS complex. Digoxin toxicity can "irritate" cells in the atria, leading to enhanced automaticity and spontaneous depolarization of this tissue and hence atrial tachycardia. Digoxin increases vagal tone on the AV node, which slows and decreases conduction down the AV node. The very high digoxin level leads to marked increased vagal tone on the AV node, and is a reason why there is only 4:1 conduction through the AV node (for every 4 atrial impulses, only 1 is conducted through the AV node down into the ventricle). When one sees atrial tachycardia with such high degree AV block, think digoxin toxicity!

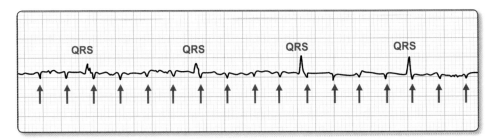

Figure 11.2　Atrial tachycardia with high degree AV block, suggestive of digoxin toxicity. Only one out of every 4 P waves (arrows) is conducted

The below rhythm strip shows an example of **ventricular flutter** (Figure 11.3). Ventricular flutter is an unstable ventricular arrhythmia that can be thought of as existing in a spectrum of ventricular arrhythmias between ventricular tachycardia and ventricular fibrillation. Ventricular flutter is an unstable arrhythmia that occurs at a rate of between 200 to 300 beats per minute. There is little organized ventricular contraction in ventricular flutter, and thus patients are often pulseless and unresponsive. The rhythm will often quickly degenerate to ventricular fibrillation. Treatment of patients with ventricular flutter is immediate defibrillation.

Take a look at this unusual ECG tracing on the following page (Figure 11.4). Not uncommonly, this will occur and the telemetry alarm will go off. While at first this appears to be some bizarre arrhythmia, on careful inspection one can see that there are normal appearing QRS complexes (arrows), distinct from everything else on the ECG tracing. This is an example of artifact, and how artifact can initially appear to be an arrhythmia. Common causes of artifact include shivering, seizure, tremor and even tooth brushing.

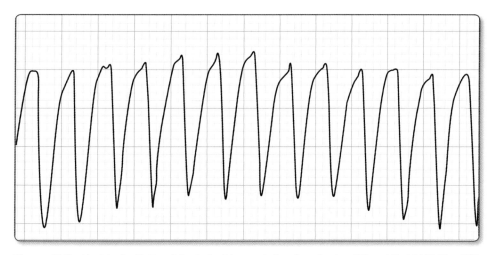

Figure 11.3 Ventricular flutter. Adopted with permission from Levine GN and Podrid PJ. The ECG Workbook. John Wiley and Sons

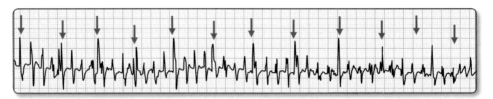

Figure 11.4 An example of an ECG tracing with artifact. Notice the larger QRS complexes (arrows) occurring at regular intervals. The smaller deflections occurring at a very fast rate are artifact

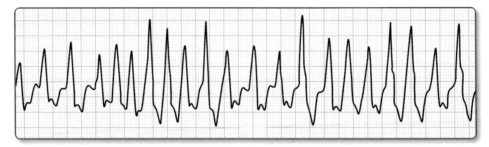

Figure 11.5 The ECG tracing that results when someone with a bypass tract develops atrial fibrillation. There is marked variation in the QRS complex morphologies and RR intervals

The above rhythm strip is an example of an unusual ECG tracing (Figure 11.5) that we mentioned before in Chapter 7. This rhythm strip shows the ECG tracing that occurs when someone who has a bypass tract (such as in Wolff-Parkinson-White syndrome) develops atrial fibrillation. The rhythm is irregular and the QRS comlexes are of varying width. The QRS impulses are of varying width because some of the impulses that reach and depolarize the ventricle travel down the AV node and His-Purkinje system, resulting in narrow QRS complexes, while some other impulses that depolarize the ventricle travel down the bypass tract, resulting in wide QRS complexes.

Sometimes, impulses traveling down the AV node and His-Purkinje system and impulses traveling down the bypass tract arrive in the ventricle at the same time, resulting in QRS complexes that are a hybrid of a narrow QRS complex and a wide QRS complex. The resulting rhythm strip is essentially a montage of narrow QRS complexes, wide QRS complexes, and QRS complexes of intermediate width. As we discussed before, patients who develop this arrhythmia should not be treated with medications that slow conduction down the AV node, as this may somewhat paradoxically lead to an increase in heart rate as more impulses travel down the bypass tract and depolarize the ventricles, and can lead the patient to develop ventricular fibrillation.

The below rhythm strip illustrates an example of what is called **ventricular bigeminy** (Figure 11.6). In ventricular bigeminy, each normal beat is followed by a **premature ventricular contraction (PVC).** Ventricular bigeminy is usually a benign arrhythmia, does not portend the development of sustained ventricular tachycardia, and usually does not require any specific treatment. Patients will usually have no symptoms or only a sensation of "skipped heart beats". In some patients with ventricular bigeminy, automated devices that measure blood pressure and heart rate may only sense the normal beats and not the PVCs, and display a very slow heart rate, only half the actual heart rate.

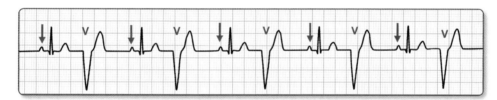

Figure 11.6 Ventricular bigeminy. After every normal P wave (arrow) and QRS complex is a premature ventricular contraction (PVC), denoted on the ECG tracing by a "V". This pattern of every normal beat followed by a PVC is called ventricular bigeminy

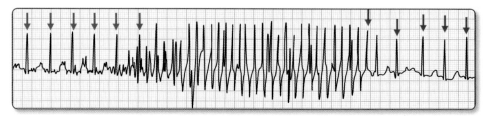

Figure 11.7   Another example of artifact. The "arrhythmia" seems to start while there are still normal QRS complexes, and normal QRS complexes are again seen immediately as the "arrhythmia" terminates. These are important clues that this is actually artifact instead of an actual real arrhythmia

The above ECG tracing is another example of artifact (Figure 11.7). There are several important keys to recognizing that this is artifact. First, in the mid portion of the ECG strip there are the bizarre narrow QRS complexes occurring at a very fast rate. Such QRS complexes are not easily explained by any real arrhythmia. Second, the "arrhythmia" seems to start while we can still see normal QRS complexes. Third, immediately upon termination of this "arrhythmia" one can see normal QRS complexes occurring. In most cases of tachyarrhythmias, when the arrhythmia breaks there is usually a short pause before normal sinus rhythm resumes. It would be very unusual to see normal QRS complexes from normal sinus rhythm occurring essentially immediately as the arrhythmia terminates.

CHAPTER 12

Basic Life Support and Adavanced Cardiac Life Support Treatment of Arrhythmias

Basic life support (BLS) and advanced cardiac life support (ACLS) are best learned through a dedicated course, such as those designed by the American Heart Association (AHA). In this chapter, we will briefly review some of the most important aspects of BLS and ACLS as it relates to the treatment of arrhythmias. In this chapter we will address three basic types of arrhythmias: (1) ventricular fibrillation (VF) and pulseless ventricular tachycardia (VT); (2) tachycardia with a pulse; and (3) bradyarrhythmias.

VENTRICULAR FIBRILLATION (VF) AND PULSELESS VENTRICULAR TACHYCARDIA (VT)

The simplified BLS algorithm for health care providers emphasizes the following steps:

1. Assess if the patient is unresponsive and not breathing (or only abnormally gasping for breaths)
2. Activate the emergency medical response system and get an automated external defibrillator (AED) or manual cardioverter/defibrillator

3. Check for a pulse. Spend no more than 10 seconds doing this

4. Begin CPR (cycles of 30 chest compressions and 2 breaths, beginning with 30 chest compressions)

5. Check for a shockable rhythm as soon as the AED/defibrillator arrives. Shockable rhythms in such settings are VF and VT. Give one shock ASAP.

The simplified BLS algorithm (Figure 12.1) is in the accompanying figure. It emphasizes cycles of good quality CPR and defibrillation (if indicated) as soon as possible.

Heartman's Clinical Pearl

Irreversible brain damage begins to occur as early as 4 minutes after the brain is deprived of oxygen, such as occurs during pulseless cardiac arrest. In patients who develop witnessed VF and cardiac arrest, survival rates decrease 7–10% for every *minute* that passes until successful defibrillation if no bystander CPR is provided. Even with bystander CPR, survival rates fall 3–4% per minute until successful defibrillation. In patients who are not successfully defibrillated within minutes of cardiac arrest, survival with intact cognitive function is dismal. Survival rates with "code blue" are much higher in patients with VF or pulseless VT who are quickly defibrillated than is survival with other rhythms (such as pulseless electrical activity or asystole). Therefore, the single key driving force when treating the patient with arrhythmia and cardiac arrest is to as quickly as possible determine if the patient is in VF or pulseless VT and to immediately defibrillate the patient.

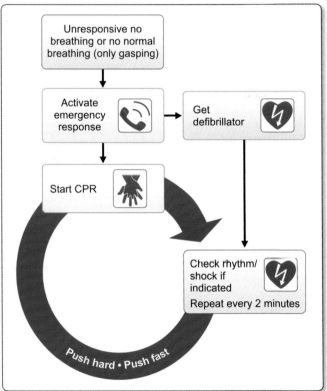

Figure 12.1 The simplified adult BLS algorithm. Reproduced with permission from Advanced Cardiac Life Support Provider Manual

A simpler form of CPR is recommended for lay persons not trained in CPR who attend to persons with out-of-hospital cardiac arrest. The simpler approach, called "**hands only CPR**", consists only of chest compressions, without stopping to administer breaths.

The ACLS algorithm for VF and pulseless VT (VT without a pulse) involves the same basic concept as the BLS algorithm of prompt defibrillation and 2 minute cycles of CPR. It additionally incorporates obtaining IV or intraosseous (IO) access to administer drugs, the administration of certain drugs, and use of an advanced airway (e.g. intubation). The initial steps in the ACLS algorithm for VF and pulseless VT include recognizing that the patient is nonresponsive, activating the emergency medical response system, obtaining an AED or manual cardioverter/defibrillator, and starting CPR. The patient should be defibrillated as soon as an AED or manual cardioverter/defibrillator is available if the rhythm is determined to be VF or pulseless VT.

In the new ACLS guidelines, as soon as the first shock is delivered, CPR should immediately be resumed and continued for 2 minutes before the rhythm is reassessed or a pulse check is performed. When IV or IO access is established, a **vasopressor** drug (one that constricts the blood vessels) should be administered. The two choices are epinephrine (1 mg) or vasopressin (40 units). After 2 minutes of CPR since the first shock, the rhythm and pulse are reassessed. If the patient remains in VF or VT, then another shock is delivered. CPR is again immediately resumed for 2 more minutes. If the patient remains in VF or VT, the antiarrhythmic drug amiodarone can be administered (the first dose is a 300 mg bolus).

A simplified version of the ACLS algorithm is presented on the following page (Figure 12.2). Key points emphasized in the new ACLS guidelines include the following:

- CPR should be initiated as soon as possible. The regimen is 30 compressions and 2 breaths
- Defibrillation should be performed as soon as possible
- Immediately after a shock is delivered, CPR is resumed for 2 minutes before the rhythm is reassessed and a pulse check is performed
- Epinephrine or vasopressin can be administered when IV (or IO) access is established. However, administration of these agents has not been shown to improve long-term outcome, and CPR and prompt defibrillation should not be delayed in order to establish IV access
- If the patient remains in VF or VT despite multiple shocks, the antiarrhythmic agent amiodarone can be administered. However, administration of neither amiodarone or of lidocaine (another antiarrhythmic agent) has ever been shown to improve long-term outcome.

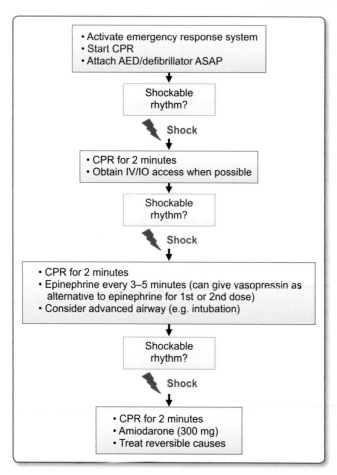

Figure 12.2 A simplified ACLS algorithm for VF and pulseless VT. Adopted with permission from Advanced Cardiac Life Support Provider Manual

TACHYCARDIA WITH PULSE

The 2010 ACLS algorithm for tachycardia with a pulse has been simplified from prior algorithms. ACLS guidelines for tachycardia with a pulse emphasize several important factors to be considered in the treatment of tachyarrhythmias:

- Assess whether or not the patient is asymptomatic or is symptomatic and unstable

- Serious symptoms and signs that would classify the rhythm as an "unstable tachycardia" and warrant urgent treatment include hypotension, acutely altered mental status, signs of shock, ischemic chest discomfort, and acute heart failure

- It is important to try to determine whether the tachycardia is a cause of the symptom or a result of the symptom and underlying medical condition

- Ventricular heart rates <150 beats per minute usually do not cause serious signs or symptoms (unless the patient has a severely reduced left ventricular ejection fraction or severe coronary artery disease)

- The approach to the arrhythmia may vary depending on whether it is a narrow complex tachycardia or a wide complex tachycardia

The ACLS tachycardia with a pulse algorithm is one algorithm that addresses both narrow and wide complex tachycardias. For the purposes of simplicity, we will divide the algorithm into two separate algorithms, one for narrow complex tachycardias with a pulse and one for wide complex tachycardias with a pulse (Figures 12.3 and 12.4).

Heartman's Clinical Pearl

The energy level used for defibrillation of VF or pulseless VT depends on whether the defibrillator delivers a "monophasic" or "biphasic" shock, as well as the manufacturer of the defibrillator. The energy level for AEDs is pre-set, so when using an AED deciding what energy to choose is not an issue. When using a manual cardioverter/defibrillator that delivers a biphasic shock, which most recently manufactured devices are, the recommended energy level is usually 120–200 joules (J), depending upon the manufacturer of the device. If the recommended energy level for defibrillation is not know, the ACLS protocol suggests that one use the maximum energy level of the device. For devices that deliver a monophasic shock, which are primarily older devices, an energy level of 360 J is recommended.

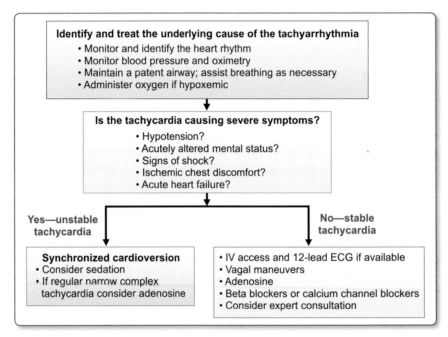

Figure 12.3 A simplified ACLS algorithm for the management of a patient with narrow complex tachycardia with a pulse. Adopted with permission from Advanced Cardiac Life Support Provider Manual

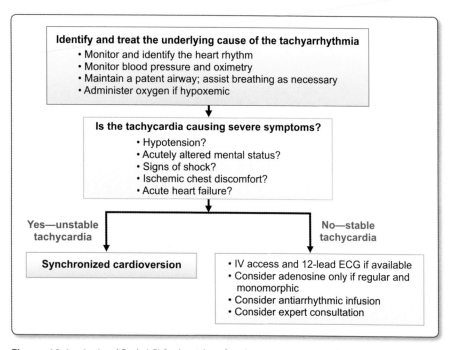

Figure 12.4 A simplified ACLS algorithm for the management of a patient with wide complex tachycardia with a pulse. Adopted with permission from *Advanced Cardiac Life Support Provider Manual*

We will first discuss the approach to a patient is a narrow complex tachycardia. The initial step in the algorithm is to identify and treat any underlying cause of the arrhythmia and to take several steps to monitor and support the patient. The next step is to determine if the tachycardia is causing severe symptoms. Treatment then depends on whether or not the tachyarrhythmia is causing severe symptoms or not.

Adenosine is a very quick-acting and short-acting drug that blocks conduction down the AV node. It is very effective for terminating AVNRT and AVRT, which as you remember are reentrant arrhythmias that both involve the AV node. It may occasionally also terminate atrial tachycardia. The initial dose is 6 mg rapid IV push, followed by a normal saline flush of 20 cc. A second dose of 12 mg can be administered if the first dose fails to break the arrhythmia. **Beta blockers** and certain **calcium channel blockers** both slow conduction through the AV node. These drugs may, therefore, also terminate AVNRT or AVRT. They will slow the ventricular response rate if the arrhythmia is atrial fibrillation or atrial flutter. They usually have little effect on the ventricular rate if the rhythm is atrial tachycardia or MAT.

The approach to a wide complex tachycardia is similar to that of a narrow complex tachycardia with a couple exceptions. Adenosine should only be considered if the patient is stable and the QRS complexes are regular and monomorphic. Adenosine might terminate the rhythm if it is a SVT (such as AVNRT or AVRT) with BBB. Antiarrhythmic treatment with agents such as procainamide or amiodarone can be considered to terminate the arrhythmia. Procainamide is infused at a rate of 20–50 mg/min until the arrhythmia terminates, hypotension ensues, the QRS width increases >50%, or a maximum dose of 17 mg/kg has been administered. Amiodarone is given as a first dose of 150 mg over 10 minutes.

The approach to the patient with a wide complex tachycardia and a pulse is given in Figure 12.4.

Heartman's Clinical Pearl

In **synchronized cardioversion**, the cardioverter/defibrillator monitors the heart rhythm (Figure 12.5) while shocking the heart, so that the shock is not inadvertently delivered to the heart during what is called the "vulnerable period" (a period of repolarization during the cardiac cycle that corresponds to the T wave). A shock delivered to the heart during the vulnerable period while the heart is repolarizing can cause ventricular fibrillation. Cardioverter/defibrillators can deliver unsynchronized defibrillation shocks to the heart using just the two "quick look" pads. However, in order to give synchronized shocks, additional leads usually need to be connected to the patient, so that the device can monitor the heart rhythm using these leads and deliver the actual shock using the "quick look" pads. You usually need to push the "synchronize" button on the cardioverter/defibrillator to tell the device that you want to deliver a synchronized shock. If the cardioverter/defibrillator is ready to deliver a synchronized shock, small triangles, squares, circles or arrows will be displayed on the device's monitor above each QRS complex, as shown in the below display. This demonstrates that the device is successfully recognizing and tracking the QRS complexes, the period in the cardiac cycle when the shock is delivered.

Rhythms such as atrial tachycardia, multifocal atrial tachycardia (MAT) and junctional tachycardia are due to enhanced automaticity of cells and not usually due to a reentrant arrhythmia. Because of this, cardioversion usually does not terminate these arrhythmias when they occur.

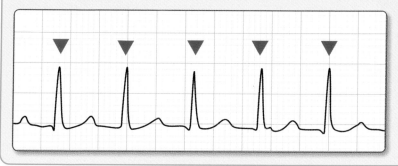

Figure 12.5 An example of the display on a cardioverter/defibrillator showing that the device is successfully tracking the QRS complexes. This particular device displays triangles above each QRS complex to demonstrate it is able to see and track the QRS complexes

BRADYCARDIA WITH PULSE

As we have discussed, there are many different arrhythmias that can cause bradycardia. The ACLS algorithm addresses the more general entity of bradycardia from any cause. Key aspects of the ACLS algorithm for bradycardia include (Figure 12.6):

- Identifying and treating the underlying cause.
- Assessing if the patient is symptomatic
- Initial treatment with atropine
- Treatment with either a medication that increases the heart rate (dopamine or epinephrine) or transcutaneous pacing if atropine treatment is ineffective
- Expert consultation and/or transvenous pacing if necessary

Symptoms that warrant acute treatment, if they are believed to be caused by the bradycardia and not some other medical condition, include hypotension, acutely altered mental status, signs of shock, ischemic chest discomfort, and acute heart failure. In such cases, the initial treatment is **atropine.** Atropine acts to decrease vagal stimulation of the heart, and thereby increases depolarization of the SA node and increases conduction down the AV node. The dose of atropine for symptomatic bradycardia is 0.5 mg IV. This dose is repeated every 3–5 minutes, up to a maximum total dose of 3 mg.

If atropine is ineffective, then the bradycardia is treated with either infusion of a drug that increases the heart rate or transcutaneous pacing. In unstable patients, particularly those with heart block, transcutaneous pacing is the first-line treatment if IV access cannot quickly be established to administer atropine. Drugs that can increase the heart rate that can be used in the setting of symptomatic bradycardia include dopamine and epinephrine. Dopamine infusion is begun at a rate of 2–10 mcg/kg/min and titrated to patient response. Epinephrine infusion is begun at a dose of 2–10 mcg/min and titrated to patient response.

The adult bradycardia with pulse algorithm is presented in the accompanying flow diagram (Figure 12.6).

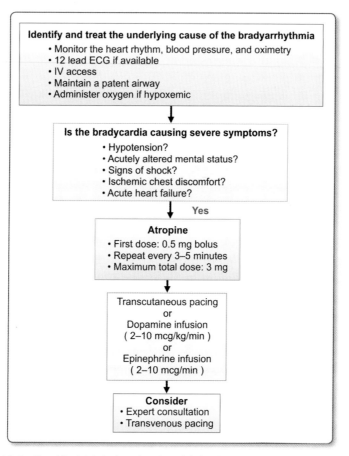

Figure 12.6 Simplified ACLS algorithm for adult bradycardia with pulse. Adopted with permission from Advanced Cardiac Life Support Provider Manual

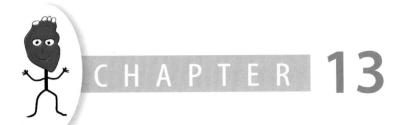

CHAPTER 13

Summary

Most tachyarrhythmias can be easily diagnosed if one takes a systematic approach to the arrhythmia. For tachycardias, we use this simple three step approach of:

1. Determine if the QRS complexes seen in the arrhythmia are narrow or wide

2. Determine if the QRS complexes are occurring at regular or irregular intervals

3. Determine if there is any evidence of P waves or atrial activity present

If the rhythm is a narrow complex regular tachycardia, there are only six possible causes: sinus tachycardia, atrial tachycardia, atrial flutter, junctional tachycardia, AVNRT or AVRT. If the rhythm is a narrow complex irregular tachycardia, there are only three possible causes: multifocal atrial tachycardia (MAT), atrial flutter with variable conduction down the AV node ("variable block"), and atrial fibrillation. Looking for P waves or atrial activity usually allows one to make the specific diagnosis of which arrhythmia is causing the narrow complex tachycardia.

For wide complex tachycardias, the rhythm in almost all cases will be either SVT with BBB or VT. Tricks that can help determine whether the wide complex tachycardia is due to SVT or due to VT include:

1. Determining if the QRS complexes are perfectly regular (in morphology and in the RR interval) or slightly irregular
2. Determining if P waves are present before each QRS complex or there is evidence of organized atrial activity (such as flutter waves), or if there is P wave dissociation (AV dissociation).

The presence of perfectly regular wide QRS complexes suggests the rhythm is an SVT, though we need to keep in mind that monomorphic VT can sometimes appear pretty regular. Slightly irregular QRS complexes favor a diagnosis of VT. Very irregular QRS complexes are usually due to polymorphic VT (though remember that atrial fibrillation in a patient with WPW can produce notably irregular QRS complexes). P waves or atrial activity before each QRS complex strongly suggests an SVT. P wave dissociation (AV dissociation) is almost always associated with VT.

Bradyarrhythmias may be due to sinus bradycardia, a junctional rhythm, second degree heart block, or third degree (complete) heart block. Looking for P waves can allow one to make the diagnosis in most cases. If the P wave rate is faster than the QRS rate, then heart block must be present.

When coming upon an arrhythmia, whether a bradyarrhythmia or tachyarrhythmia, one should always look carefully to see if pacer spikes are present. Sinus tachycardia with a paced ventricular rhythm can easily be mistaken for a wide complex tachycardia if one does not notice the small pacer spikes at the beginning of the QRS complexes.

ACLS algorithms emphasize the importance of activating an emergency medical response system, quickly obtaining an AED or manual cardioverter/defibrillator, initiating high quality CPR, prompt cardioversion if the patient is unstable, and immediate defibrillation if the patient is pulseless. Remember, brain death begins within minutes in the pulseless person with VF or VT, and immediate defibrillation is paramount.

We have now finished your introductory course on arrhythmias. You should now have a basic understanding of what causes arrhythmias, where and how they occur in the heart, and how to diagnose and treat them. Heartman and I congratulate you on a job well done!

INDEX

Page numbers followed by *f* refer to figure

A

Abnormal
  depolarization of the heart 4
  heart rhythm 8
Accessory bypass tract 28
Advanced cardiac life support 81, 82f, 84f, 86f, 87f, 91f
Agent, antiarrhythmic 83, 84f, 86f, 91f
Algorithm, ACLS 83
Amiodarone 83
Antidromic conduction 29, 30f
Apixaban 22
Arrhythmias
  basic types of 81
  life support treatment of 81
  ventricular 77
Artifact 77
Asystole 7
Atrial
  arrhythmias 11

fibrillation 8, 11
flutter 8, 17f, 18f, 41, 43f, 46, 47
tachycardia 5, 8, 11, 14, 41, 42, 44, 46f, 48
Atrioventricular node 23
AV
  dissociation 51, 52f, 53
  nodal reentrant tachycardia (AVNRT) 5, 9, 23, 24, 26f, 41, 42
  nodal tachycardia (AVRT) 5
  reentrant tachycardia 23, 24, 25, 28

B

Beats, skipped heart 79
Beta blockers 19, 22
Beta-adrenergic stimulation 4
Bigeminy, ventricular 79, 79f
Block, variable 45, 46f, 92
Bradyarrhythmias 6, 55, 70, 81
Bradycardia 6
Bundle branch block (BBB) 48

C

Calcium channel blockers 19, 22
Cardioversion, synchronized 89
Cardiovert 19, 81, 83
Catheter ablation 27
Causes of
  arrhythmias 5, 10
  tachyarrhythmias 6, 10
  bradycardia 6
  sinus bradycardia 56
  tachyarrhythmias 5
  heart block 61, 62, 63, 64, 65, 69
Complex
  irregular tachycardia 41, 46
  regular tachycardia 40, 41, 44, 45, 46
  tachycardia 41, 48, 50, 54, 73
Contraction, premature ventricular 79
Coumadin 22
CPR, hands only 83

D

Dabigatran 22
Defibrillation 33, 81, 83, 89
Deflections of the ECG baseline 47
Depolarization of
    AV node 7
    ventricular tissue 7
Development of atrial fibrillation 21
Devices, automated 79
Diagnosing
    arrhythmia 52
    bradyarrhythmias 66
    persistent sinus tachycardia 12
    tachyarrhythmias 38
Digoxin 19, 22
Discomfort, ischemic chest 85
Diseases
    coronary artery 33, 37, 85
    heart 27
    intrinsic SA nodal 56
    ischemic heart 27, 31
    lung 16
    structural heart 27
Dropped beat 60f, 61

E

Ectopic junctional tachycardia 24
Eliquis 22
Enhanced automaticity 4, 5, 10, 13, 32

F

Failure, acute heart 85
Fibrillation, ventricular 36, 36f, 37, 81
Fibrillatory waves 20
First degree heart block 59
Flutter, atrial 92
Flutter, ventricular 77, 77f
Flutter waves 17

G

Generating a depolarization 1

H

Heart block develops 6
Heart's pacemaker 3
His-Purkinje system 2, 7, 24f, 28f, 30f, 50, 54, 57, 59, 63

I

Impulses
    depolarization 70
    electrical depolarization 70
    pacemaker depolarization 72
Intervals, regular or irregular 92
Intraosseous 83
Irregular ventricular response rate 20

J

Junction of the atria 57
Junctional
    escape rhythm 62, 63f, 64, 65, 69f
    rhythm 7, 57, 58, 67
    tachycardia 4, 9, 23, 24, 41, 42, 43, 44, 45, 65

L

Left atrial appendage 19, 21
Left bundle branch (LBB) 1, 2
Lidocaine 83

M

Major causes of tachyarrhythmias 38
Mobitz
    type I second degree heart block 59, 60, 67f
    type II second degree heart block 60, 67, 68f
Monomorphic VT 34
Multifocal atrial tachycardia 4, 8, 11

N

Narrow QRS complex 38, 50, 57f, 63f
Node
    AV 70, 72
    SA 70, 72

Nonconducted
    beats 59, 60
    impulses 59
    P wave 60*f*, 61*f*, 62*f*, *67f*, *68f*
Nonparoxysmal junctional tachycardia
    24
Non-reentrant junctional tachycardia 24
Non-sustained VT 34
Normal
    depolarization of the heart 1, 2
    sinus rhythm 1

O

Orthodromic conduction 29

P

P wave dissociation 51, 52*f*, 53*f*, 65
Paced rhythms 70
Pacemaker implantation 57, 60, 61, 64
Pacemaker of the heart 57, 62, 63
Pacing, AV sequential 74
Parts of the heart involved in tachyarrhythmias
    9
Polymorphic VT 34
Pradaxa 22
Premature

atrial contraction 27, 31
    ventricular contraction 27, 31
Pulmonary vein ablation 21
Pulse, tachycardia 81, 85
Pulseless VT 33
Purkinje fibers 2

Q

QRS
    complex 38, 41*f*, 42, 44, 46, 48, 50, 51, 53,
        56, 58, 59, 60, 61, 63, 65, 66, 67, 69,
        72, 73
    intervals 49
    morphologies 48, 53

R

Rate, heart 70
Reentrant
    circuit 4, 5, 10, 13, 17, 33
    loop 17
Rhythm
    atrial paced 72
    defibrillator monitors the heart 89
    heart 70
    paced 70
Right bundle branch (RBB) 1, 2

Right bundle branch block (RBBB) 48
Rivaroxaban 22

S

SA node 1
Second degree heart block 59, 68
Sinoatrial node 1
Sinus
    bradycardia 55, 56*f*, 57*f*, 66
    tachycardia 8, 11, 41*f*, 44, 48, 51*f*, 72
Spikes pacing 72
Spikes ventricular pacing 74
Stable VT 33
Support
    advanced cardiac life 81
    basic life 81
Supraventricular tachycardias 8
Sustained VT 34
Syndrome
    sick sinus 75
    tachybrady 75

T

Tachyarrhythmias originating
    atria 11
    ventricles 32

Tachycardia
    atrial 89
    multifocal atrial 89, 92
    narrow complex 85
    narrow complex irregular 92
    pulseless ventricular 81
    unstable 85
    wide complex 85
Terminates, atrial fibrillation 75
Third degree heart block 62
Thrombus 19
Torsades de pointes 32, 35
Tracing, ECG 77, 78f, 79f
Triangles, particular device displays
    89
Triggered automaticity 10

U

Unstable
    patients 90
    tachycardia 85, 86, 87
    ventricular arrhythmia 77

V

Variable
    block 46, 47
    conduction 46
Vasopressor drugs 83
Ventricular
    arrhythmias 32
    escape rhythm 63, 64, 65, 69

fibrillation 10, 32, 36
rhythms 7
tachycardia 4, 5, 8, 10, 29, 32

W

Warfarin 22
Wave, P 70, 92
Wide
    complex tachycardia 92
    QRS complex 38, 48, 50, 51, 63
Wolff-Parkinson-White (WPW) syndrome 4, 28

X

Xarelto 22